Homestead Cows

THE COMPLETE GUIDE TO RAISING HEALTHY, HAPPY CATTLE

ERIC RAPP AND CALLENE RAPP

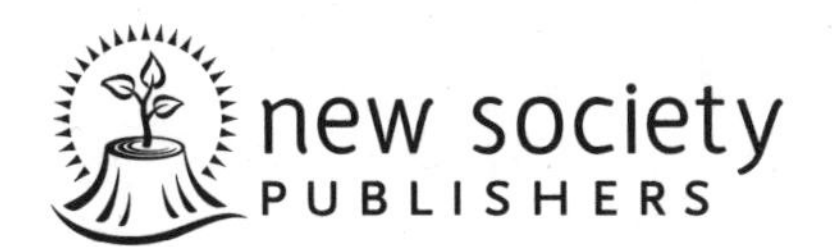

Cover design by Diane McIntosh.
Cover photos: ©iStock. Bottom left supplied by Eric Rapp.
Unless otherwise noted, all photos and illustrations by Eric Rapp.

Printed in Canada. First printing June, 2021.

Any other inquiries can be directed by mail to

New Society Publishers
P.O. Box 189, Gabriola Island, BC V0R 1X0, Canada
(250) 247-9737

LIBRARY AND ARCHIVES CANADA CATALOGUING IN PUBLICATION
Title: Homestead cows : the complete guide to raising healthy, happy cattle / Eric Rapp and Callene Rapp.
Names: Rapp, Eric, 1959- author. | Rapp, Callene, 1965- author.
Description: Includes bibliographical references and index.Identifiers: Canadiana (print) 20210169168 | Canadiana (ebook) 20210169176 | ISBN 9780865719477 (softcover) | ISBN 9781550927405 (PDF) | ISBN 9781771423366 (EPUB)
Subjects: LCSH: Cattle.
Classification: LCC SF197 .R36 2021 | DDC 636.2—dc23

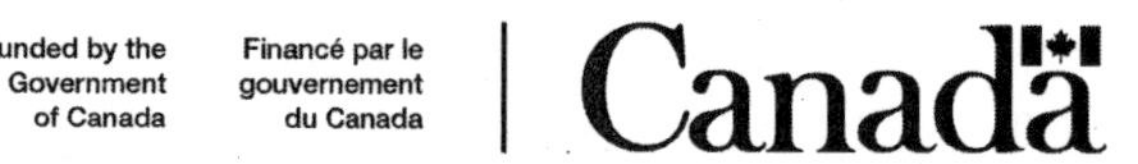

New Society Publishers' mission is to publish books that contribute in fundamental ways to building an ecologically sustainable and just society, and to do so with the least possible impact on the environment, in a manner that models this vision.

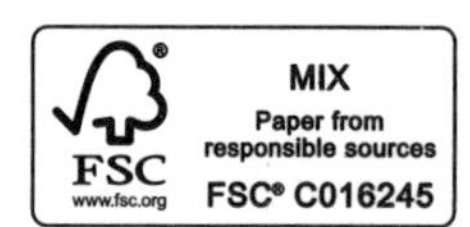

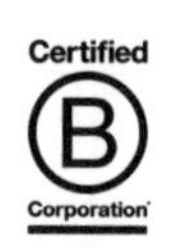

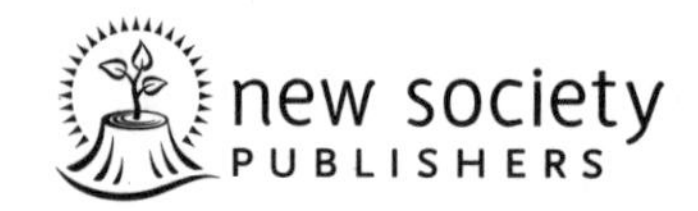

Contents

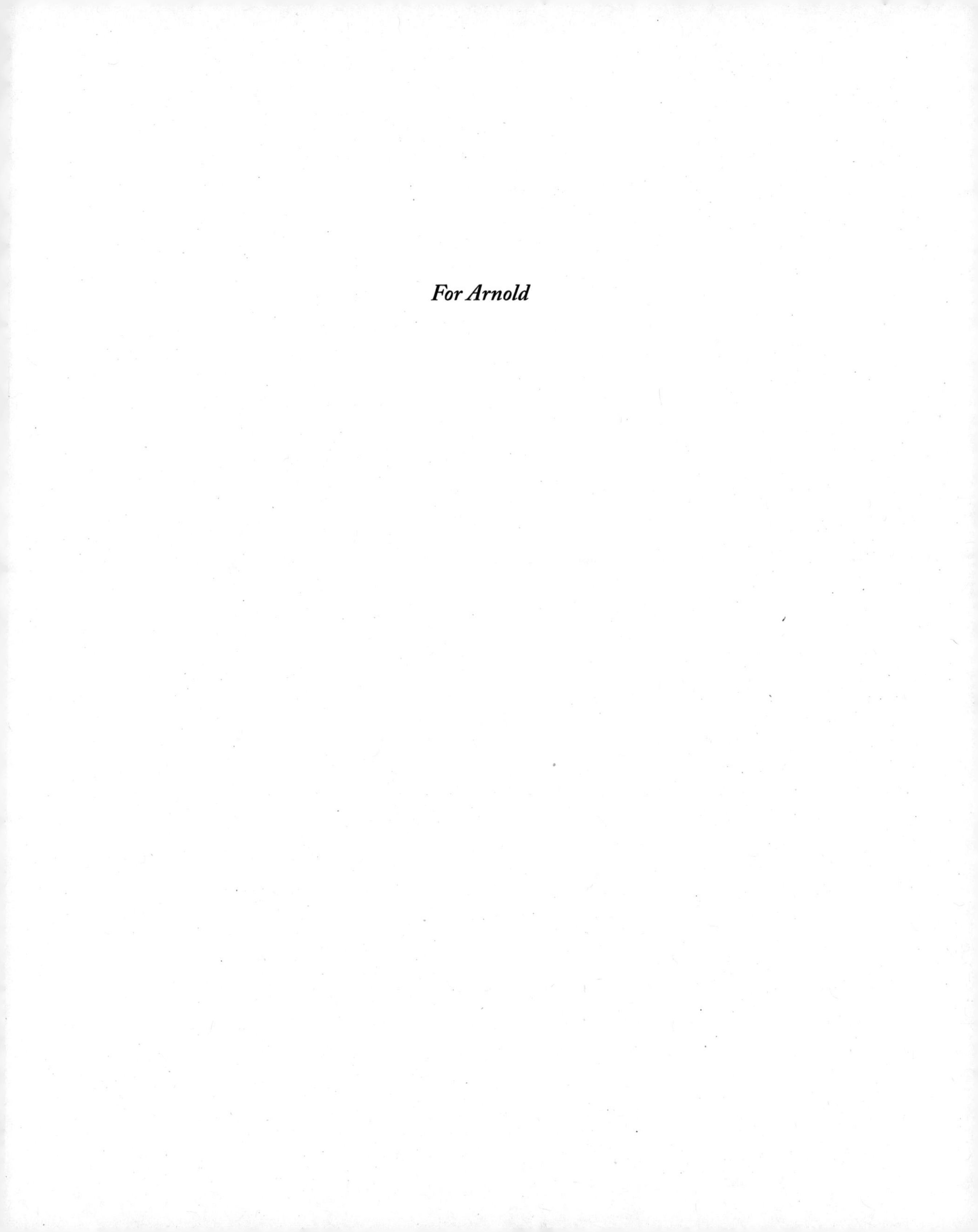

For Arnold

Acknowledgments

While writing may be a solitary pursuit, making a book definitely is not. Thanks to the folks at New Society Publishers for making this book happen. Thanks to Emily for all her photographic contributions and moral support; and thanks to Ian, who edited this book into cohesiveness. As people whose organizational style can best be described as "There appears to have been a struggle," we appreciate how you folks all helped to keep us on the straight and narrow, and we hope to work with all of you again on future endeavors.

—Callene and Eric Rapp
Kansas, February 2021

Introduction

If you've picked up this book, I'm guessing and hoping that you're already interested in getting cows, or a cow. Congratulations! Cows were one of the best decisions we ever made for our farm.

When I submitted the first draft of this book to the publisher, the editor pointed out that it really needed a section on "Why should people get cows?"

I was floored. I mean, why *wouldn't* people want cows?

But he was correct in that there is a lot to think about before taking the plunge into cattle ownership, and like any livestock decision, it should not be taken lightly.

No livestock of any kind is labor free. They will need things like feed and water on a regular basis, and they will need it when the weather is 112°F (44°C) or when it's –12°F (–24°C) and snowing. They need it in the dark before and after work, and often at the time least convenient to you. Taking on the responsibility of owning livestock, especially larger animals such as cows, means putting their needs and well-being above your comfort many times, but they give us so much more in return. And, while (once again) no livestock is labor free, a cow contentedly grazing on well-managed pasture comes pretty close at times.

Cattle can, over time, improve your land and soil. The soil we have now is a result of millions of years of synergistic efforts between animal, plant, and microbe. Degraded soils can be improved by careful management of cattle and pasture. It would seem a shame to have cows just for the land improvement benefits and not take advantage of their other good qualities, but soil improvement alone is reason enough to have grazers on the grass.

Another key benefit to having cattle is a deeper understanding of the human–animal connection. We have evolved with animals as our companions, our responsibility, and our source of food. It is a profound thing to truly understand that the circle of life is indeed a cycle, and each element plays a part in nourishing and being nourished. The notion that there can be food of any type without sacrifice is an artificial construct of a society that has drifted too far away from the basic understanding that every life consumes something.

And probably one of my favorite reasons to have cows: cows are cheaper than therapy. Being around a group of placidly munching cattle can't help but lower your blood pressure, and they never repeat your stories… at least, not to human ears. What's said in the pasture, stays in the pasture.

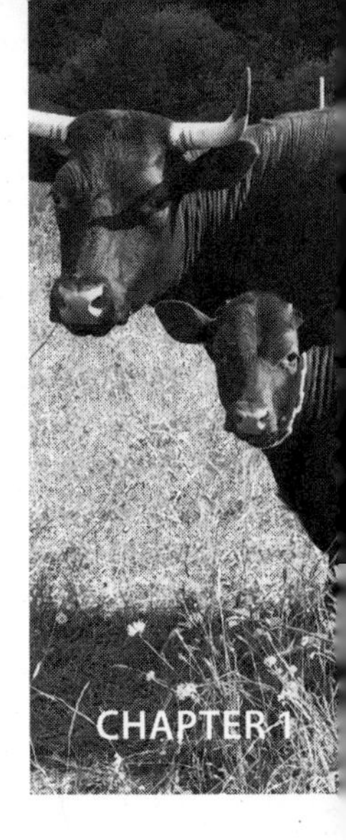

Humans and Cattle

A Brief History of Cattle

Cattle evolved from a prehistoric bovid called an Aurochs (*Bos primigenius*) that roamed Europe for several million years.

Aurochs were huge compared to our modern cattle, some standing 5 feet or more tall at the shoulder. Fossil records show some variability depending on the geographic region and time period they were found in, but Aurochs are believed to have regularly weighed over 3,000 lbs.

Hunting Aurochs was a primary activity for prehistoric humans, and a dangerous one. The Aurochs lacked the easygoing nature of the modern bovine, to say the least. Cave art shows the Aurochs winning the contest regularly.

Approximately 8,000–10,000 years ago, several domestication events took place nearly simultaneously in the Fertile Crescent region in the Near East and in the Indian subcontinent. Fossil records show that the massive Aurochs gave rise to our modern cattle, both the humpless European *Bos taurus* and the humped Zebu type, *Bos indicus*. While each is considered a separate species, *Bos taurus* and *Bos indicus* are capable of interbreeding and producing fertile offspring.

Early uses of domesticated bovines included milk and draft power, as well as meat. Some of the earliest pottery artifacts have been found to have milk residue. Fermented milk products, such as yogurt and cheese, have been dietary staples as long as humans have interacted with bovines. Indeed, much of the history of human civilization is written in tandem with cattle.

The Aurochs has the distinction of being one of the only progenitors of a species to exist at the same time as its descendants. As their habitat dwindled, Aurochs became fewer and fewer, and ultimately the last one died in Poland in 1627. Interestingly, a project has begun to attempt to re-create the Aurochs and install it in some of its ancestral grazing grounds, helping to manage abandoned farmland and retain biodiversity by keeping forests from overtaking the land.

Cattle in the United States

Cattle came to the New World early in the European settler exploration phase. Historical documents have Columbus bringing a few cattle as work animals on his second voyage in 1493, and as travel to the new world increased, more cattle were delivered. By 1512, the West Indies had a thriving livestock industry.

Spanish cattle began to be imported in the early 1500s began spreading from Florida through the southeast into the southwest and from Mexico into Texas. British cattle were brought to Jamestown in 1611.

Early use of cattle in the US was primarily for hides and tallow; the beef was more of a byproduct and often discarded because of the lack of adequate storage and transportation. There was no selection for beef quality at the time.

In the early 1800s, to feed the growing urban market, cattle were driven on the hoof to urban centers and processed there. These are the romantic cattle drives of the era from 1845 through 1865.

The invention of the refrigerated rail car made it possible to ship the beef, not the beef animal, and the number of cattle on western ranches doubled between 1880 and 1890.

The Shift to Feedlots

Feedlots began appearing in larger numbers in the 1950s. Their rise was driven by a new consumer preference (with the income to back it up) for marbled meat, which occurs when cattle are fed grain; low grain prices, coupled with subsidies; and the development of antibiotics, which allowed more animals to be confined in closer quarters, without disease becoming rampant.

In 1935, the USDA reported that 5.1% of the 42.8 million cattle were in feedlots. By 1963, 66% of cattle were grain fed, and of those 40% were in feedlots.

Packing houses followed the feedlots, and in the 1960s IBP (Iowa Beef Producers) began packaging cuts of beef such as steaks and roasts into what is called "boxed beef," rather than shipping the primals to butcher shops and the butcher breaking them down into individual cuts. This boxed beef increased the efficiency of shipping meat, as boxes could be packed more effectively than large sides and primals, and it increased the foothold of the feedlot industry.

In the modern beef era, 85% of beef production is controlled by four companies. And the cattle have grown, too. In 1975 the average dressed weight of cattle was 579 lbs., and in 2016 the average was 817 lbs.

A huge shift in how cattle are raised has occurred in less than a century. Like a pendulum swinging as far as it can one way, we have moved completely away from how cattle were raised just a couple of generations ago. Cattle are now judged largely on how big they can get, how much they can produce, and how fast they can do it, with little regard for the impact on the animal or the environment.

Fortunately, when a pendulum swings one way, eventually it has to swing back. Consumers are becoming more educated about the health benefits of grassfed beef and dairy products. Grassfed beef counted for sales of $272 million in 2016, versus just $17 million in 2012, and at the time of this writing, sales were doubling every year.

Even better, a growing number of people are taking the plunge and beginning to consider raising their own beef, and making their own dairy products.

And that is where you and this book come together.

What's Your Plan?

Assessing Your Needs... and Your Wants

What is your ultimate goal when adding cows to your farm? A small home dairy? A freezer full of good-quality beef? Adding some income to your farm?

All of those are fantastic goals, but each requires a slightly different mindset and plan.

Meat and milk don't have to be mutually exclusive. A milk cow bred to a beef sire can provide a calf that, while it might not be competitive in a feedlot, can provide an ample supply of meat for a family.

And, as a cow will need to be bred and have a calf regularly in order to produce milk, so you can have a calf going into your freezer on an annual basis.

It's not instantaneous, though. Cattle take time to mature. That calf will spend a good couple of years growing (and eating) before it reaches harvest size.

And dreaming about homemade cheese is great, but there is a lot that goes into preparing before you get to that point. How much cheese do you want to produce on a regular basis? Do you have a place to store and age cheese? If it takes roughly five quarts of milk (depending on fat content and type of cheese desired) to make a pound of cheese, at what point are your facilities overloaded with cheese? Or, will you have enough milk on a regular basis to produce what you want and need?

A lactating cow needs to have that milk removed from her udder daily or sometimes multiple times daily, depending on the cow. Either you need to do it or her calf needs to do it. Will you or someone in your family be able to keep up with that commitment? Or should you make a milk share plan with the calf? Cattle are relatively easy to care for compared with other livestock, but they thrive on consistency.

How much milk do you actually need? A dairy breed cow can produce gallons of milk daily. And a dairy breed that produces multiple gallons of milk might produce too much milk for both you and her calf. Other livestock can benefit from excess milk and the byproducts of cheese making; pigs and chickens both love and can make use of the excess. But that cow still needs to be milked out daily.

Cattle can also be a terrific source of income. Purchasing calves in the spring, grazing them in the summer and then selling them in the fall can be a good source of revenue, provided the market cooperates. Are you willing to take a loss, or would you have the resources to hold on to them until the market turns around?

Sample Vet Services and Prices

Service	Range of Fees
Travel Charge	Usually so much per mile, from a base rate of about $50 up to $100, depending on the distance
Castration	$35–$75 depending on age and size
Pregnancy Checking	$10–$20 per head
Vaccines	$8–$10 per injection
Health Certificate	$25–$50
Examination	$45–$60

How many cows do you want? Better yet, how many cows do you have room for? Hopefully we will answer that question later in the book, but cattle are large animals. They thrive best when they have room to move around. Since cattle are physically bigger than other livestock, there are some differences in managing them.

Many "rules of thumb" say you need one to two acres per cow, but that doesn't mean you can plunk a cow down into an acre lot and be done with it. Less space equals more management, and very few small acreages will allow for year-round grazing. Most climates will have some times of the year when you will need to feed hay. There are some folks raising cattle who are able to "stockpile" winter forage by leaving pastures ungrazed part of the year, but this takes a larger acreage that most of us have access to.

Unlike pigs, which can be fed on a variety of feeds, or goats, which benefit from browsing and prefer it over grazing, cattle depend on having grass, or forage in some form. There are a variety of types and means of getting forage: pasture, hay, silage, etc. Make sure you know what's available to you and what the cost will be before you go get cows. Do you have a place to store your hay and keep it from the weather? Large round hay bales are meant to be stored outside, but small square bales need shelter. Many hay producers will deliver hay, but prefer to do a large load at a time to maximize their efficiency and factor that cost into the price per bale. One or two bales will more than likely mean an extra delivery charge.

Transporting cattle is more effort than smaller livestock. And, at some point you will have to transport them, whether it's home when you buy them or to the processor when it's time to harvest them. Goats and sheep can hitch a ride in a minivan, but adult cattle will need some sort of trailer or livestock rack to move anywhere.

Do you have a large animal vet close by? If so, the time to develop a relationship is before you have a problem. Vet fees can vary from region to region. A good cattle vet might be hard to find, as it seems as though many newly graduated veterinarians are going into small animal practice, leaving a lack of vets with large animal expertise.

Regulations! No one likes them, but they do need to be considered. Are large animals allowed on your property? Is your plan to create a home business around your cow and her products? Regulations regarding the sale of raw milk and raw milk products vary by state. Even if that's not in your plan, check into what you can and can't do before you start. Needs and plans change, and it's nice to know what your options can be before you get in too deep.

Where is your beef processor located? If beef is in your plan, how far away is the nearest processor? Is it state or federally inspected? Custom slaughter facilities can process only for the owner of the animal. You can split ownership of the cow between families, and each gets their share of the meat and the processing costs, but it is not legal to sell the meat retail.

Research your beef markets. If your goal is to sell to restaurants, the meat will need to be USDA inspected, and being able to supply a restaurant with the quantities of specific cuts they need can be challenging.

What about you and your family? Is everyone on board with helping take care of the cow, or cows? They may be relatively low maintenance, but all livestock require food, water, and shelter—no matter what season it is.

Is everyone on board knowing that the calf they spend two years naming, raising, and seeing every day is going to wind up on the dinner table? Kids are resilient, thank goodness, but life is going to be much easier if everyone is on the same page beforehand, or at least knows what book they're reading from.

Cattle need shelter from the elements. This does not mean they need to be kept in a fancy barn, but, at minimum, they need shade in the summer and protection from the wind and rain in the winter. As we will see later, cattle can tolerate a variety of temperature and environmental situations, but some care must be taken to provide for extremes.

Also, a catch pen near that shelter is a good idea because your cow will know when you need to have her at a certain place at a certain time… and she'll be sure to be at the opposite end of the pasture and not interested in your agenda.

Shelters for cattle can be very basic, and using repurposed materials can make them as close to free as possible.

And, while the cow herself might not need an enclosed barn, consider the humans in the equation, too. If you plan to milk year-round, an enclosed barn will be greatly appreciated by the milker during extreme weather.

Some of the best advice I ever got was never to plan a barn or shelter in the summer when it's dry. Plan it during the winter months or the rainy season to see just where water or snow collects, where the wind blows hardest, or just how wet your future barn site may get. Watch the rain runoff to make sure you aren't planning it right where water runs through or collects. The warmth of summer often makes those wet, nasty days a faint memory… but they will come back eventually.

As far as costs go, the biggest expense will be the initial purchase price of the animals. Cattle can range in price from a few hundred dollars to tens of thousands. While in most instances you do get what you pay for, depending on the circumstances, that expensive cow might not be much better than the one you barter with your neighbor for. Be wary of cattle that seem too cheap. There's usually a reason.

These are some of the questions people getting into cattle should ask themselves well before they purchase that first cow. My sincere hope is that the chapters following will help you answer those questions for yourself, and make the most informed choices you can as you start your cattle adventure.

Breeds and Cow Selection

CHAPTER 2

Breeds of Cattle

CATTLE SERVE A MYRIAD OF PURPOSES in our world, more than just milk or meat. Draft power has been an important part of our history with cattle, and, yes, settling the west would have been more difficult without the hardy and patient ox.

Breeds as we know them today developed from the specific needs of humans, the environment, and to a certain extent from the cattle themselves. There are breeds that excel at milk production, some that excel at meat production, some that are very good at both, and some that are very good at both with the added bonus of making splendid oxen teams.

As we read earlier, cattle evolved from a common ancestor into the two species we know today, *Bos indicus* and *Bos taurus*. The array of today's highly unique breeds of cattle are all subunits of one or the other of those two species. No matter how wildly different a Highland cow looks from a Holstein, when bred together they will produce viable, fertile offspring. In fact, *Bos indicus* cattle and *Bos taurus* cattle can also be successfully bred, which is what gave rise to the modern Brahma cattle.

There are literally hundreds of breeds of cattle in the world, each developed to fill a certain need or environmental niche. It would be the subject of an entire book in itself to discuss all of them, so here I've only tried to profile a few that I have had some experience with over the years, or ones that are known to be easier for novice cattle owners to work with.

Don't let this list limit your search. Check out the rest of the breeds on The Livestock Conservancy's Conservation Priority List; ask around at different agricultural events; and talk to people who have worked with a breed that catches your attention. Be aware, however, that each breed has superfans who will extol the virtues of their favorite and may gloss over the negative. There is no one perfect breed; just choose one that will work well for you in your particular situation. And be honest with yourself about both your experience and your facilities.

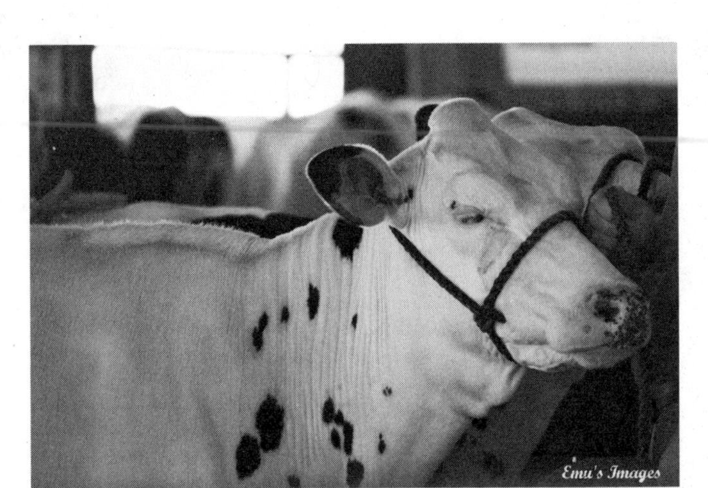

Holstein cow.
CREDIT: EMILY NYMAN

Dairy Cattle

Holstein

If you are looking for the ultimate dairy breed, Holstein cattle are the first to come to mind. Their black-and-white color pattern has become the symbol for what most of non-rural America thinks cattle look like. The majority of dairies in the US milk Holstein or Holstein cross cows.

Holsteins of superior genetics, with the proper nutrition and husbandry, have been recorded producing 72,000 pounds of milk over the course of a year. That's

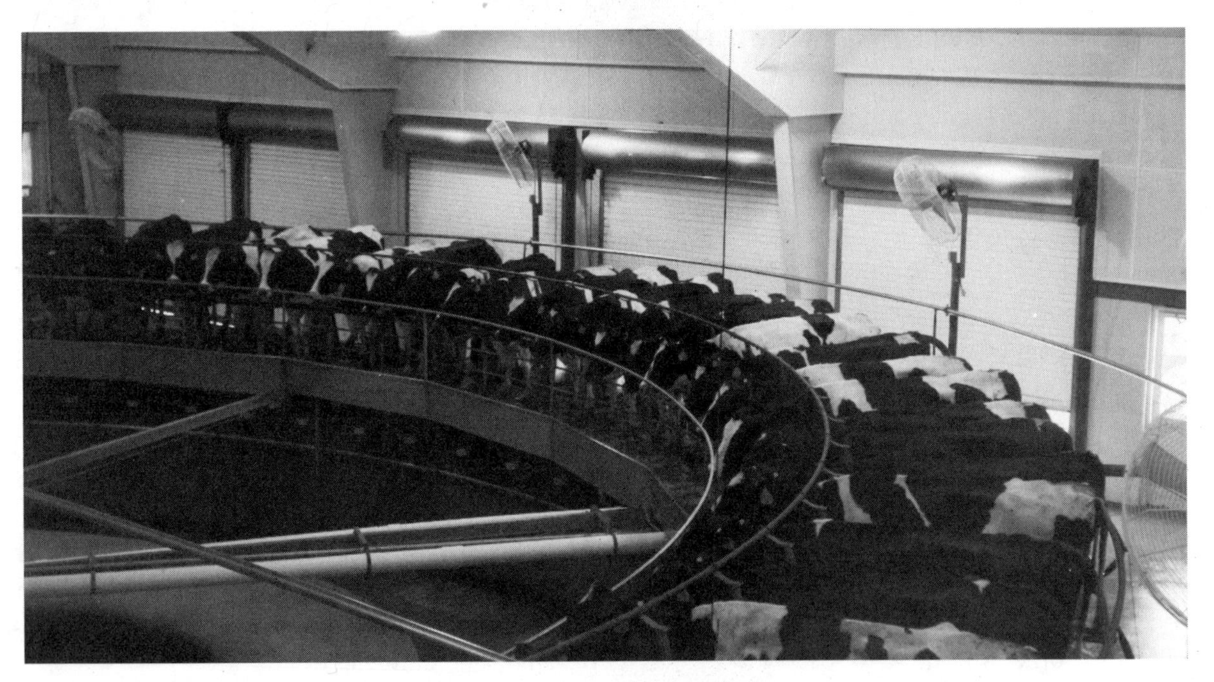

Holsteins in a dairy.

9,000 gallons in a year, or over 24 gallons *per day*. That's much more than the average of 23,000 lbs./ 2674 gallons per year, 9 gallons per day.[1]

Most of us will never run across a high-producing Holstein, but even 8 gallons per day might be more than the average family is interested in for their own use. On the other hand, because they are fairly common, Holsteins are one of the easier breeds to find.

Holsteins are of Dutch origin and often known by their historic name of Holstein-Fresian for the geographic area the breed originated in. The first Holstein in America landed in Boston in 1852.

No breed has been as affected by advances in genetic selection, artificial insemination, and modern technology as the Holstein. Unfortunately, while the advances have been great, there has been a down side. The Holstein breed as a whole has begun having difficulty with inbreeding issues, thanks to the overuse of certain sires. Fortunately, the same technology can help correct problems within the breed, if used wisely.

Holsteins are large cattle, with mature cows weighing an average of 1,500 lbs. They are born with horns but are typically dehorned due to the close quarters they are generally managed under. They have the lowest milk fat percentage of any of the common dairy breeds: 3.65 %. (As volume goes up, milk fat content goes down.)

Brown Swiss

Brown Swiss are one of the most beautiful of dairy cattle breeds, and also possibly one of the oldest. They are typically a light brown, almost grayish color, although they can range from nearly white to dark chocolate brown. As you might suspect from the name, the breed originated in Switzerland, and some historians estimate they might have been present there as early as 4000 B.C.

Their milk is higher in fat and protein than Holsteins', though they still produce a respectable volume, an average of 23,000 lbs. of milk in a 305-day lactation cycle. (A gallon of milk weighs 8.6 lbs., so that's 2,674 gallons of milk, nearly 9 gallons a day over 305 days.) The ratio of fat and protein in their milk results in it being superb for making cheese.[2]

They are large cows, females weighing 1,300–1,400 lbs., and most are horned, although a polled strain has shown up as well.

They are noted for having an exceptionally easygoing temperament, and are also noted for being structurally correct, long lived, and hardy. They will produce in the herd well into their teens.

My experience with Brown Swiss bears this out; one I knew lived to an astonishing age of 22, although she had stopped calving some years prior. Easygoing in any circumstance, she could be used for the littlest child to pet without fear. Despite her quiet nature, she was the top cow in the herd for years, and after her death the herd took some time to sort itself out.

Jersey

The light-brown, dark-faced, doe-eyed Jersey is the second most popular dairy breed. Their color can range from a light tan, almost gray, to an almost black color. A true Jersey will always have a black nose, surrounded by a nearly white muzzle. Their milk is the richest, highest in butterfat and protein. They are a smaller framed cow, around 800 lbs, and can produce 14,000 lbs of milk per year. They are a much more efficient cow to feed and known for having a good temperament and for calving ease. Less than 1% of heifer Jersey cows have difficulty calving, compared to 8% for Holsteins.[3]

Their richer milk and relatively efficient foraging ability makes them the cow of choice for a lot of cheese makers. They also provide a decent beef carcass.

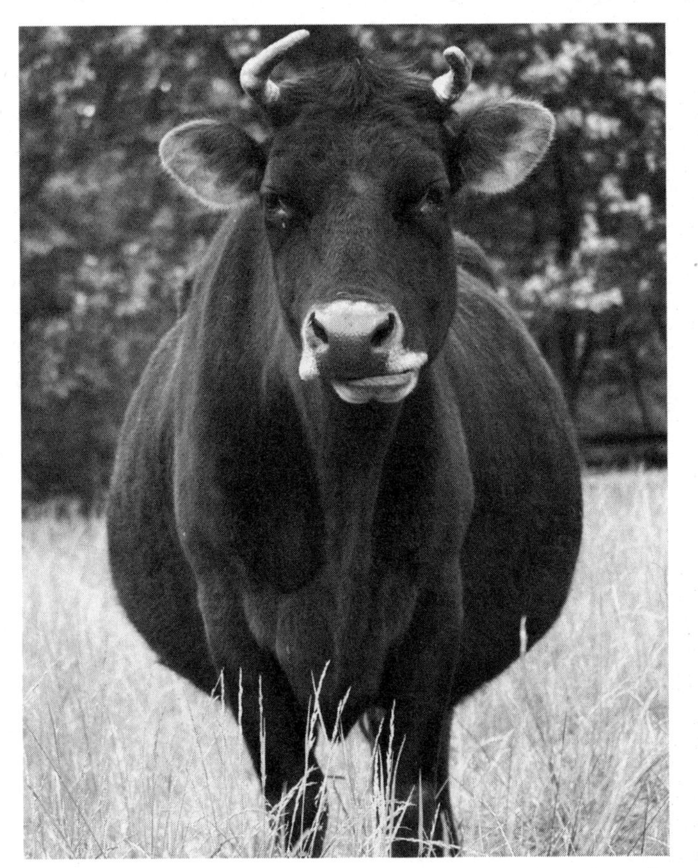

Jersey cow. CREDIT: EMILY NYMAN

Guernsey

Both Jersey and Guernsey cows originated in what is now English territory, on the Channel Islands, small islands just off the coast of Normandy.

Guernseys are medium-sized cows, slightly bigger than a Jersey but smaller than a Holstein, averaging around 1,200 lbs. They are a beautiful golden tan-and-white cow and are known for producing milk that is more yellow in color than that of other breeds. This yellow color comes from a higher level of beta-carotene in the milk, which is a precursor to Vitamin A. They are known as "Golden Guernsey" for this reason. Their milk fat and protein levels are higher, and the Guernsey's milk is considered excellent for making cheese.

They are docile and rarely flighty and are also known for having minimal calving issues.

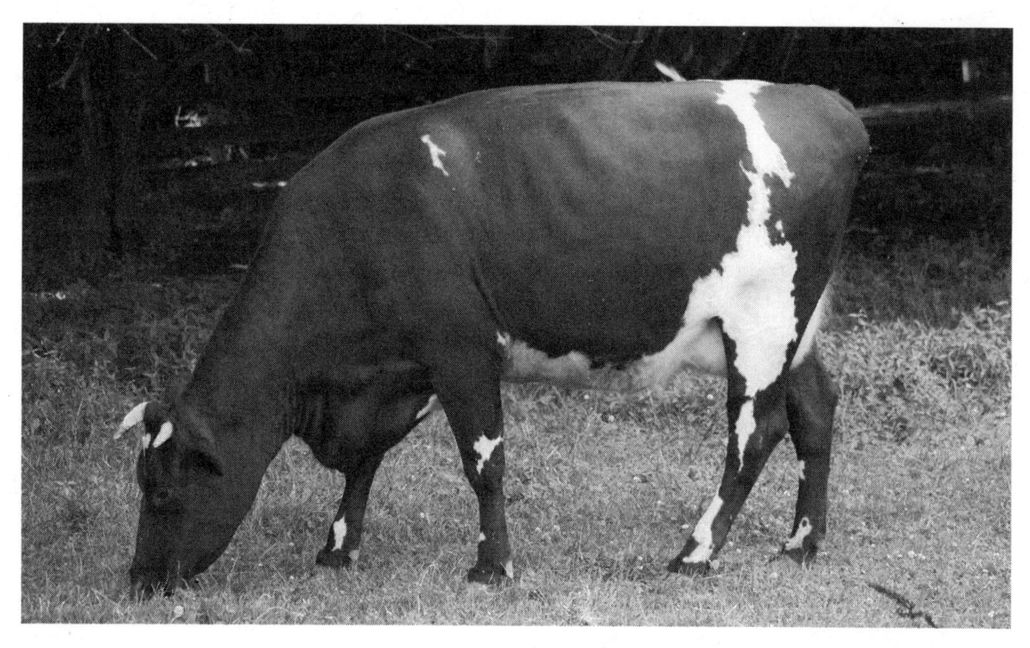

Shorthorn cow.
Credit: Emily Nyman

Shorthorn

Shorthorn cattle have the distinction of being one of the first breeds of cattle to actually be selected for certain characteristics and were first really developed in the 1600s in England.

Shorthorns are versatile, and this versatility contributed to their success with early American settlers. They provided meat and milk, and many Shorthorns pulled a plow or a wagon as well. Shorthorns come in three colors—red, white, and roan, or some combination of the three.

A polled variant was common in the Shorthorn, resulting in a strain of Shorthorns that were, well… hornless. The polled strain became very popular.

Until the early part of the 20th century, the Shorthorn was a dual- and triple- purpose breed, but specialization led to the development of dairy and beef shorthorns, and the Beef Shorthorn has been developed as a separate breed.

Milking Shorthorn cattle can produce up to 15,000 lbs. of milk per year, and they do well on forage-based dairy systems.

Native Pure Shorthorns are a subset of the Milking Shorthorn breed that have not had any of the Australian Illawara Shorthorn blood introduced, and Native Pure Shorthorns are a conservation priority for The Livestock Conservancy.

Shorthorns are hardy, calve easily, wean large calves, and have an ideal disposition for a family farm.

Beef Cattle

Angus is the most common breed of beef cattle in the US. They are popular because beef producers like the uniform black color, but they also have been selected for fast growth and for carcass traits that fit modern consumer preferences. Hereford cattle are a close second in popularity to Angus, and the perennial crossbred offspring of the two, the black whiteface cattle, make up the majority of cattle in feedlots. Both breeds and the black whiteface (also called black baldy) cattle are good beef animals and easy to find. But there are a host of other breeds to consider.

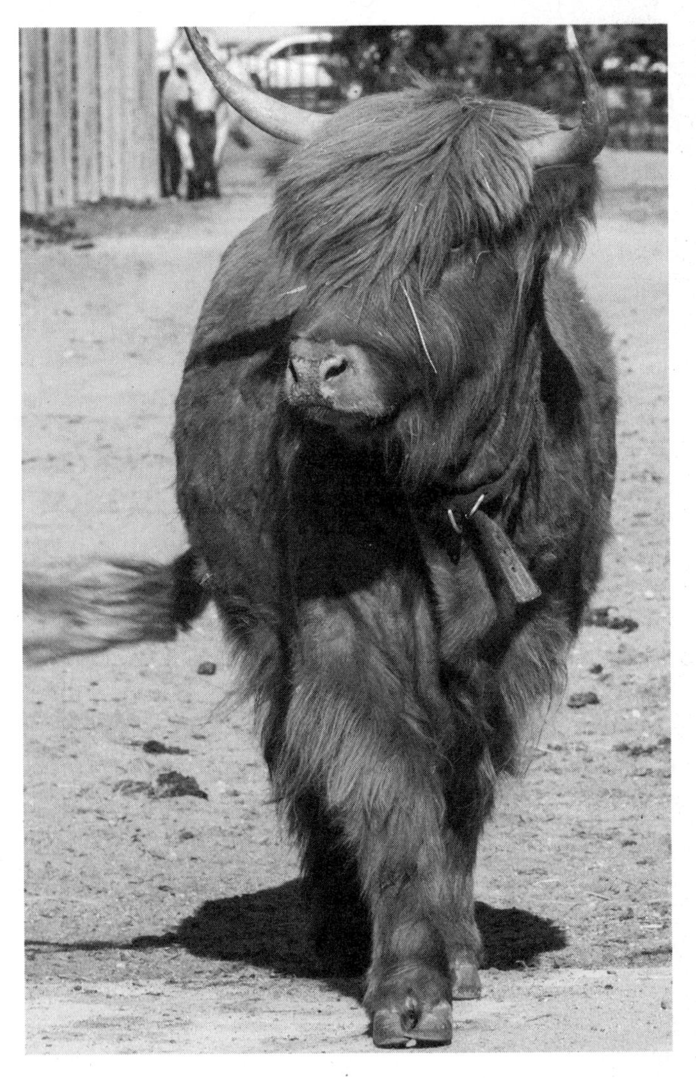

Highland cow.
CREDIT: LOU ALEXANDER

Highland

The shaggy look of the Highland cow evokes images of its native Scotland and the rugged region from which it hails. The Highland is a breed shaped by its environment and geographic isolation rather than intentional selection by humans. The Scottish Highlands have been home to these cattle for hundreds of years.

Highland cattle are hardy and long-lived, have a good reproduction rate, and make good mothers. Their shaggy double coat gives them an advantage in cold climates, but they can adapt enough to live in warm climates by shedding their inner coat while keeping the shaggy outer coat.

Highland beef is known for its tender, flavorful, and marbled characteristics. They are efficient grazers and do well on pasture-based systems. They are also known for their willingness to eat less-than-desirable forage such as forbs and weeds, and they have been used in projects to reclaim grasslands.

The Highland is one of the few pure breeds of cattle that have had no outside blood introduced, making it a unique genetic resource. They are a medium-sized breed, with cows weighing between 900 and 1,300 pounds and bulls up to 2,000 pounds. They come in a variety of colors, including white, black, red, dun, and brindle.

The breed is known for its docility, a result of its long history of close contact with humans. Animals with poor dispositions were eliminated quickly. Highland calves are small but vigorous, and dystocia, or calving difficulty, is rarely a problem. Even bulls are generally quiet and laid back.

Red Poll

The Red Poll is a dual-purpose breed from England and was developed in the early 1800s. It's named after its dark red color and the fact that it is naturally polled, or without horns. Red Poll cattle were brought to the US in the 1880s and quickly became valued for their efficient dairy production and longevity.

Although selected for both meat and dairy purposes, they have been especially prized for their quality of beef in the US since the 1960s. They excel in producing beef in pasture-based systems, and though calves are born small, they grow quickly.

Crossbreeding represents a danger to the breed, though, as the Red Poll risks being lost to commercial herd owners who want to capitalize on the breed's vigor. Red Polls need to be maintained in purebred herds as well. They are noted for their docility and even temperament and, like most cattle, respond well to gentle, consistent handling. Cows average around 1,200 pounds and bulls 1,800 pounds. They are an early-maturing breed, and can produce a choice carcass at about 14 months of age.

Milking Devon

One of the oldest purebreds in the world, the Milking Devon traces its ancestry back to the cattle of the southwestern peninsula of England, the Devonshire area, hence the name. Noted for being hardy yet active, nimble, and easy to handle, they were an easy choice for a 1623 voyage across the Atlantic Ocean.

Ox team in winter. Credit: Andrew Van Ord

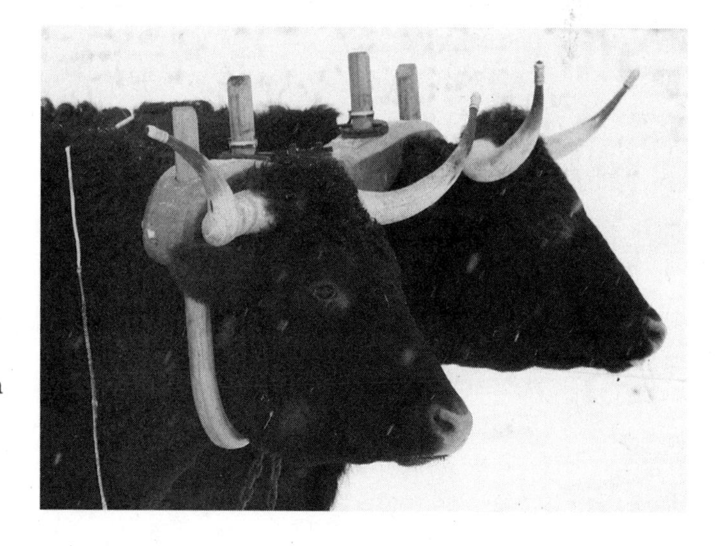

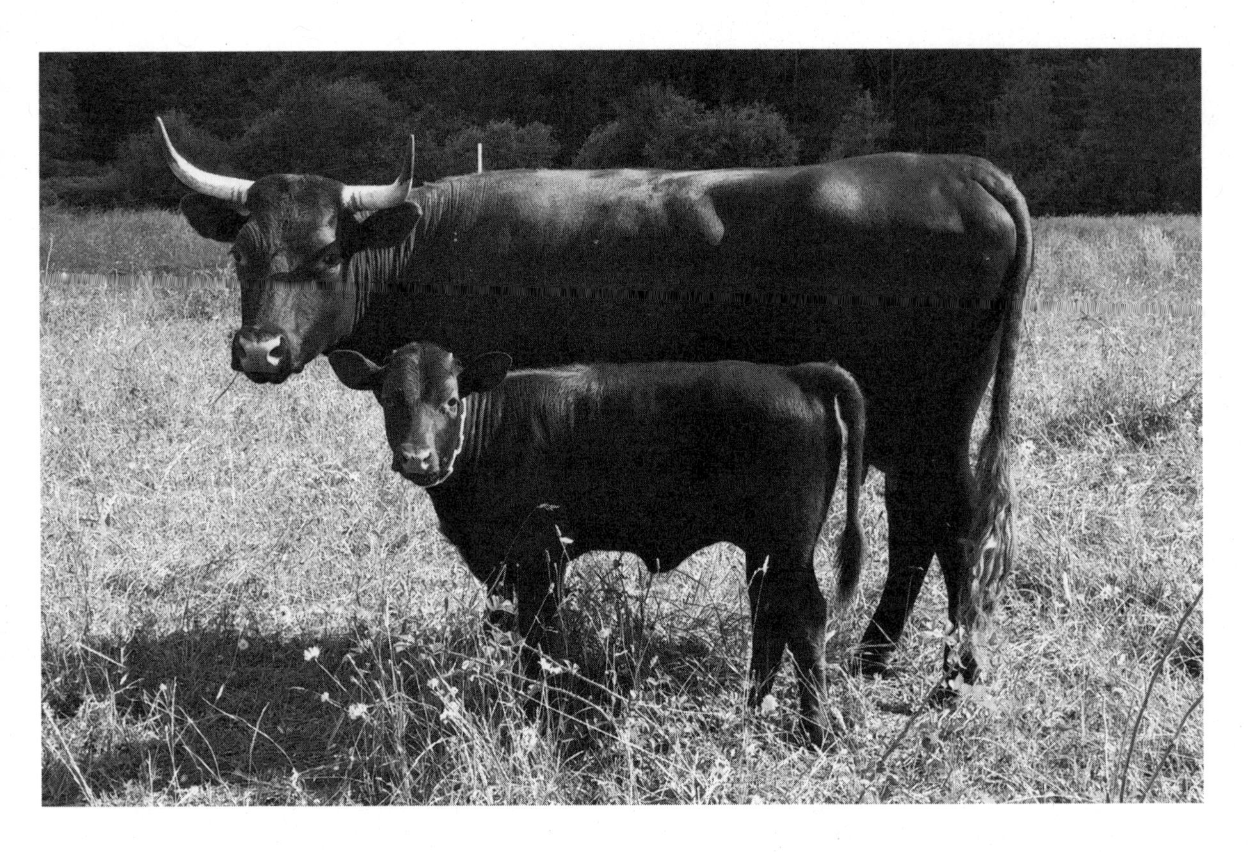

Milking Devon cow and calf. CREDIT: ANDREW VAN ORD

A bull and three heifers made the trip from England to the American colonies and formed the Milking Devon breed we know today. The breed is now extinct in England.

Valued for their ability to produce lean meat and rich milk, Devon cattle were also prized as oxen, and were widely regarded as some of the finest draft animals in the world.

By the early 1900s, though, the Devon was rarely found outside of New England, where it was still heavily favored for its production qualities and draft power. In the 1950s, the original breed organization split into two groups, the Beef Devon and Milking Devon associations.

The Milking Devon is known for its ability to produce good-quality beef and milk on marginal forage and is a breed known as an easy keeper. Their milk is around 4% butterfat. Cows will average around 1,100 pounds and bulls around 1,600 pounds, their smaller size being suitable for farms with less acreage. They are intelligent docile cattle, and they respond well to quiet handling.

Belted Galloway

The Belted Galloway is native to Scotland, from the southwestern hill country. This rugged terrain called for cattle that were hardy and easy keepers. The breed was formally developed in the late 1700s and, while selection was made for a more standard appearance, the cattle retained their maternal ability, forage efficiency, and high-quality beef. Galloway cattle are solid colored, mostly black, but the belted variant developed from the same strain. While the Beltie, as it's fanciers call it, is a separate breed from the Galloway cattle, it remains quite similar. Both grow a shaggy coat in the winter, and are very cold tolerant. The shaggy outer coat sheds water well, and the softer undercoat holds in body heat. They have hair around their ears that helps prevent frostbite. They are naturally polled and known for their docile temperaments, as many of the heritage breeds are. Their striking belted pattern is a showstopper. The most popular color is black, but they are also found in red and dun colors.

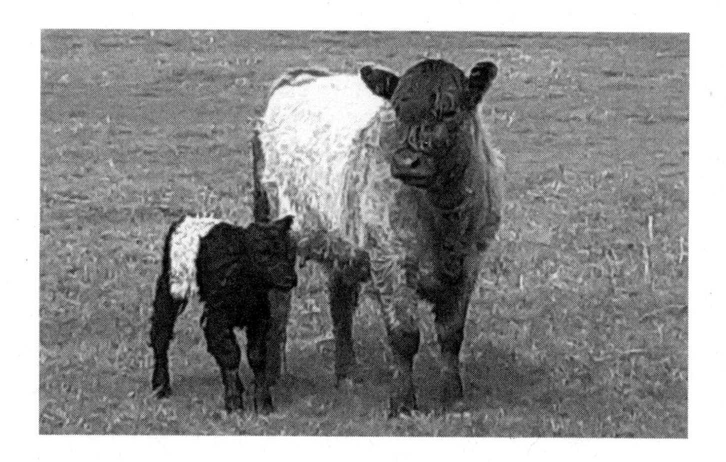

Belted Galloway and calf. Credit: Karen Thornton

Milking Shorthorn

At one time the Shorthorn was the most widely recognized breed in agriculture and one of the first to become a true breed. One of the most famous Shorthorns in history is the Durham Ox. In 1806 at 10 years of age, he weighed in at 3,500 pounds. This drew much attention from those hoping to capitalize on meat and milk production.

The Shorthorn was initially brought to the United States in the late 1700s, and remained predominantly in the Ohio and Kentucky area until the late 1800s, when the breed's popularity spread throughout the rest of the country.

The Shorthorn has always been considered a triple-purpose breed—for beef, dairy, and draft power. However, some choose this breed primarily for meat production while others select for milk production. This division was reflected when the breed association split into two groups in the early 1900s: Beef Shorthorn, or Shorthorn for beef production, and Milking Shorthorn.

Known for being good in low-input, grass-based dairy systems, efforts have been generated to locate and preserve the unimproved Milking Shorthorn. They thrive in pasture-based dairy systems, and even though the focus is on dairy, they still produce high-quality beef. They are a medium to large cow, with females weighing between 1,200 and 1,400 pounds, and bulls up to 2,000 pounds.

They can produce upwards of 13,000 pounds of milk during each lactation, and the milk is a respectable 3.3% protein and 3.6% butterfat.

Milking Shorthorns are known for their docile disposition and tractability, making this the breed of choice for oxen production in organizations like Tiller's International.

Pineywoods

Pineywoods, along with their "cousins," the Texas Longhorn and the Florida Cracker, are breeds descended from Spanish cattle brought to the New World in the early 1500s. They are collectively given the name "criollo" cattle, a term borrowed from Spanish and meaning "of European origin, but born in the New World."

Pineywoods were shaped by the environment of the Southern United States, primarily the long leaf pine forests of Alabama, Mississippi, and Georgia. Cattle were expected to get along with little human intervention or selection, resulting in a breed that is long lived, heat tolerant, and resistant to disease and parasites. Ironically, this hardiness nearly resulted in the Pineywoods becoming extinct, as they were crossed with more recent European breeds with the intention of "improving" the cattle in the south, and very few purebred cattle were kept.

Fortunately, a few families kept purebred Pineywoods herds, resulting in several unique strains, which bear the names of the families that raised them for generations. Many of these strains come with their own unique histories, which have fortunately been preserved as well.

Pineywoods are small, rugged cattle, with the angular appearance one would expect from extremely heat tolerant cattle. Cows weigh 600–800 lbs., and bulls 1,000–1,200. They can come in any color or pattern, although in some instances particular strains are noted for certain colors or patterns. Their calves are small but vigorous, and cows give birth easily.

Breed and Environment

Different breeds developed in particular environments, with traits that helped them thrive in those environments.

While it's possible to successfully raise a hot-weather-tolerant breed in a cold climate, you will need to invest substantially more in resources to keep welfare at a decent level than you would if you had chosen a breed more adapted to a cold climate.

It can be done, for sure, but it can be done better if you spend a little time thinking about what your environment is going to throw at your cattle.

Temperament

Temperament is one of the key components to consider when deciding on a breed, or an individual cow. My experience has been that most of the heritage breeds, especially those on TLC's CPL (The Livestock Conservancy's Conservation Priority List) are known for having a good disposition. Many of these breeds were developed naturally because they fit a particular niche, whether it be environmental or production, not because someone went out and decided to build a breed with X characteristics. Very little, if any, effort initially went in to creating a uniform appearance, color, or other traits of that kind. There simply wasn't time.

When you depend on animals for your livelihood, you need animals that can get along without much intervention from you. And, by the same token, you don't have time or patience to put up with ones that are mean, flighty, or aggressive. Those traits do exist and may have their purpose, but not for a small holder with young children who will be doing much of the work involved in daily care of the animals.

So put a little thought into your experience level, environment, and who will be doing the day-to-day care of the cattle—and be honest about your situation. It will make life easier in the long run.

Where to Get Your Cattle

One of the best places to purchase cattle, especially if you are new to them, is from a breeder, especially if there is a particular breed that has captured your fancy. Breeders have a substantial investment in their animals and can tell you both the ins and outs of the breed and what you can expect from their particular animals.

Purebred breeding stock will most of the time be the more expensive choice, but it can be worth it in the long run.

If you are set on a particular breed, it may not be available locally to you, especially in the case of heritage or rare breeds.

It's no secret that we are huge advocates of heritage breed cattle, and we always recommend The Livestock Conservancy as a resource for people looking for a particular breed and also as a good resource for scientifically sound information on breeding and genetics.

They also publish a breeders directory free to members, and have online classifieds to help link potential customers and sellers together.

If there is not a particular breed that catches your eye, a neighbor who has cattle might be a good potential resource, if the type of cattle they have coincides with your needs and goals.

One of the last places I would recommend getting cattle is the sale barn. Yes, you can buy cattle for years from the sale barn and never have an ounce of trouble, but it takes only one bad situation for things to get expensive really quick.

The cattle at the sale barn may have come from a place where the animals are well cared for and perfectly healthy. But once at the sale barn, they mix with every other animal that has come through. There is no way for a sale barn to clean and disinfect between each lot of cattle, and the potential for an animal to pick up a problem is great.

Often people take cull cattle to the sale barn, cull cattle that might be healthy but not be up to the breed standard. They may also be nonreproductive, or have other problems not visible to the naked eye.

If the sale barn is the only option available to you, take some precautionary measures.

If you have cattle at home, quarantine newcomers for 30 days. Have your vet come out and do blood tests to see how healthy they are and check for any diseases. Do a fecal test for parasites, and deworm if necessary.

I know one individual who brought animals home only to discover they carried Johne's disease. This ultimately led to him having to dispose of all his ruminants.

Not a fun way to enter into your cattle adventures.

Selecting Breeding Stock

One of the key phrases you always hear when talking about breeding animals is that they look "masculine" or "feminine." Other than aesthetics, there is some sound biology to go with both of those words.

In hoofstock herds, the male's job is not only to breed females, but to defend his harem from other males and from predators. To that end, he needs to be able to present an impressive display of his attributes, enough to stand up to challenge or at least to discourage rivals from attempting a challenge. A breeding male needs to be robust enough to get the job done, breeding multiple females in a short window of time.

So, there is definitely a reason for a bull needing to appear masculine.

A bull should have wide shoulders, a thick neck and a coarse head. Wide shoulders and a thick neck give him power when sparring with rivals, and a coarse head has strong bone to back it up during a challenge. A strong front end enables him to mount and breed successfully.

A bull should be muscular. Not just blocky like a feedlot steer, but the muscle should be well defined. A muscular bull will have a well-functioning endocrine

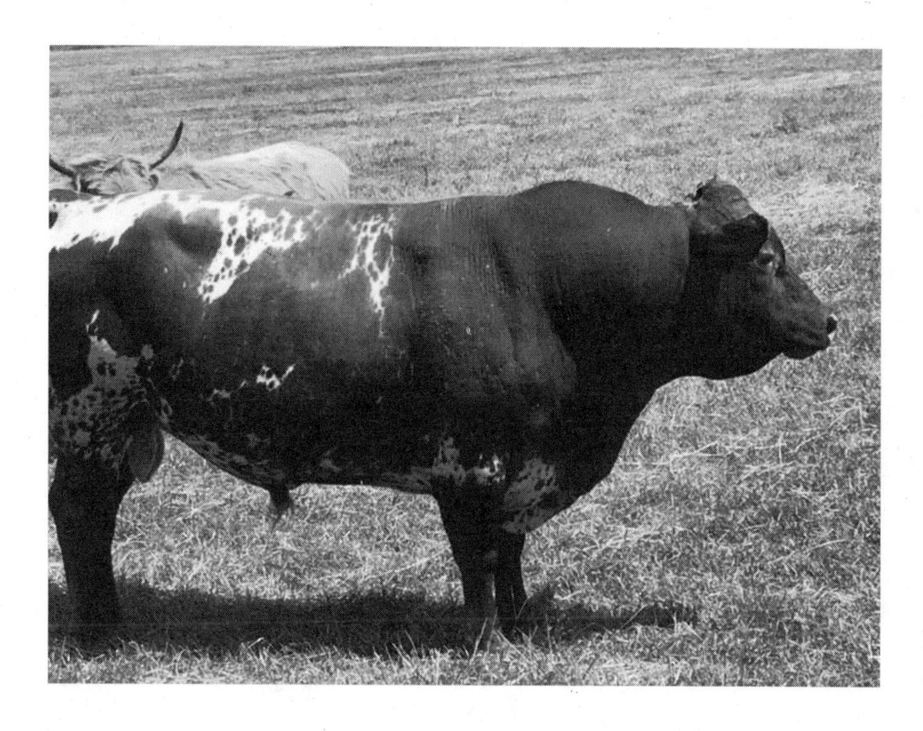

Pineywoods bull.
Credit: Hank Will

system and be at a higher level of fertility than a less muscular animal. He should have a wide chest and a deep heart girth. A bull's power is in his front end, and his appearance should reflect that.

He should have good, correct legs that are not too straight. Overly straight legs will, in the long term, not stand up (pun intended) as well as legs that are set well under the bull.

Both testicles should be the same size. If one is smaller than the other, this may be a sign of an infection or other fertility issue. The scrotum in a fertile bull should have a "buckskin" appearance and be covered with short, sparse, fine hair that will protect it from the elements and not retain heat. In hot weather a bull's testicles will descend away from his body so they don't get too hot. Elevated temperature is very hard on spermatozoa. Likewise, in winter they will be held closer to the body to stay warmer.

A cow should look feminine, which is a result of her reproductive hormones functioning properly. In contrast to a bull, whose power is in his front end, a cow's power is in her back end. A cow should have wide hips, and deep hindquarters. Her front end should be sleek, and the largest proportion on her should be her gut. A large gut capacity will allow her to eat a hefty amount and so be able to

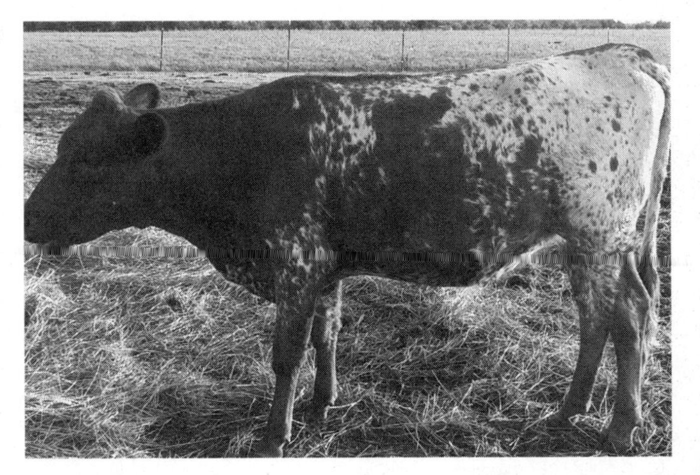

Pineywoods heifer.

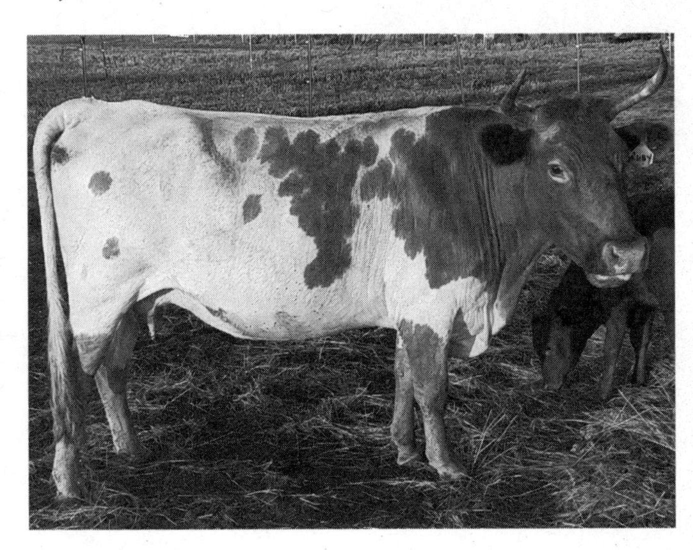

Adult Pineywoods cow.

supply nutrition, both for herself and for her calf.

Her udder should be well formed, attached close to her body in the case of a beef cow. A dairy cow, due to increased milk production, will have a larger udder, but it should still not be pendulous, which is an invitation to injury. Teats should not be too small or too large. Large teats will be difficult for a calf to nurse from.

Health Papers

When transporting cattle across state lines, a health certificate of veterinary inspection is required. Some states require a permit; all require some form of permanent identification, such as a tag or a tattoo.

Movement into and out of some states was restricted at one time, but with brucellosis being all but eradicated, and all 50 states sharing the same brucellosis-free status, this has gotten much easier.

Tracking movement of cattle between states allows monitoring of disease outbreak and can help keep a small outbreak from becoming a major one.

1 Holstein Association USA, *https://www.holsteinusa.com/pdf/fact_sheet_cattle.pdf*

2 Brown Swiss Association, *https://www.brownswissusa.com/Breed/BrownSwissBreed/BreedAttributes/tabid/175/Default.aspx*

3 "Why Jerseys," USJersey, *https://www.usjersey.com/Portals/0/AJCA/2_Docs/WhyJerseys2013.pdf*

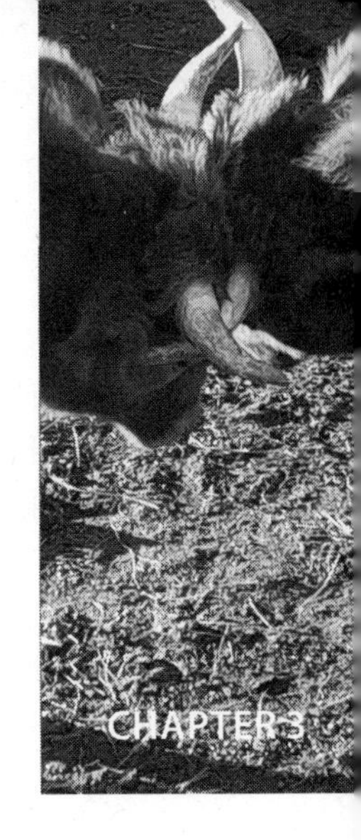

Handling, Transportation, and Infrastructure

Working Safely Around Cattle

Cattle are normally placid, gentle creatures, who prefer grazing and napping in the sun over just about any other activity.

With that said, they do possess the size, power, and equipment to seriously hurt a human being if you do not know how they think and are not prepared to relate to them in terms they can understand.

In my experience, no cow (with the exception of breeds and stock that are bred to be aggressive) will go out of her way to hurt you. Most injuries come from being in the wrong place at the wrong time, not understanding how cattle think and react, not paying attention to what the cow is communicating, or trying to force a cow to do something that she isn't interested in doing, for whatever reason.

Cattle are herd animals. That herd instinct is probably one of the key reasons cattle have adapted to domestication so well. They have a social structure with a clear leader, and once the hierarchy is established, each cow knows her place. This is not to say that the lead cow cannot be challenged for her place, but most of the time it's more than the rest of the herd wants to bother with.

Cattle will always prefer to be with other cattle if the opportunity exists. A single cow can adapt quite well, however, as long as the interactions she gets from her humans are positive. Cattle will ultimately regard people as their herd.

However, people need to be very careful that they are able to "speak cow" in order to understand the cow, understand what she is communicating, and give a clear and appropriate response. It's not fair to expect the cow to understand us; we need to be able to relate to her in terms she can understand.

Temple Grandin

Temple Grandin is a professor of Animal Science at Colorado State University.

She is also autistic and, in my opinion, has done more to improve the welfare of livestock than any other human being on the planet. She credits her autism with her being able to see the world as animals see it, and, fortunately for us and for the animals, she has been able to translate this knowledge into handling techniques and facility designs that make handling livestock easier and safer.

Livestock slaughter is an inevitable part of having farm animals in a production situation. By understanding how livestock think, see, and want to move, Grandin's slaughter facility designs have reduced the stress of moving animals through the facility to the point that it is as stress free as possible. Animals do not have a fear of death per se; what they do fear are strange smells, shadows, people moving loudly and abruptly, and pens and chutes that do not allow them to move without bunching up and being forced and pushed.

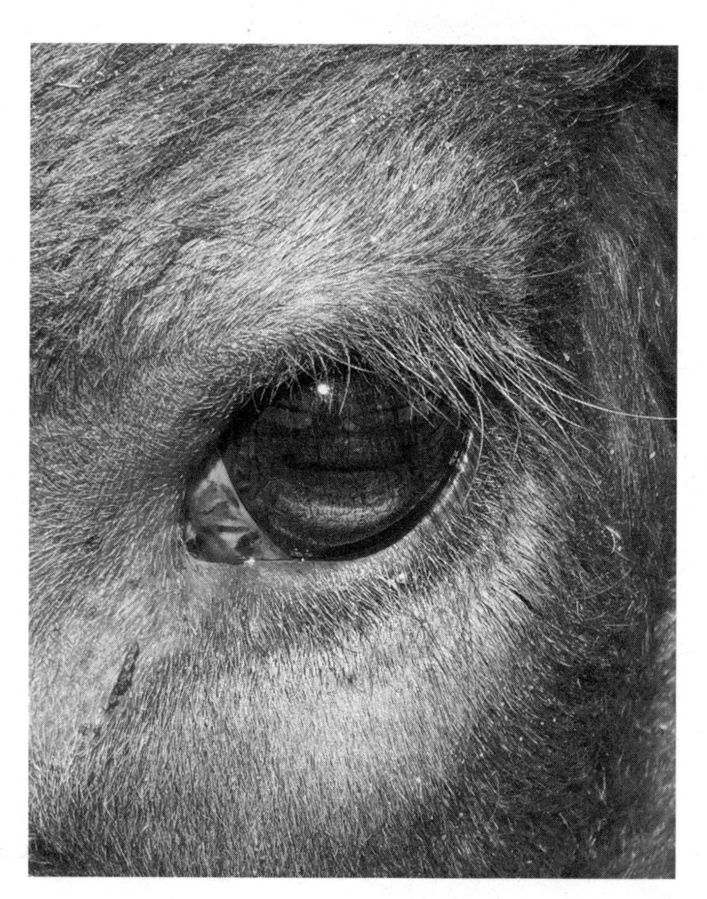

Bovine eye with horizontal pupil.

If you have not read her *Guide to Working with Farm Animals*, that should be the next book you read after this one, and, again in my opinion, it should be required reading before getting livestock of any type.

In the meantime, here are a few important points to consider.

Set your cows up to succeed, and don't blame them if you didn't.

Be quiet. Cattle hear quite well. There is no need to yell at them when you want them to move, and all the anger and volume in your voice will do is convince them something is wrong and they need to get the heck out immediately.

Cattle have a nearly 360 degree range of vision thanks to eyes wide set on their heads. This allows them to see almost a full circle, except for right behind them, and right under their noses.

This does, however, limit their depth perception. They have to adjust by raising and lowering their heads to see where they are going. If you are moving them someplace unfamiliar, letting them take a few seconds to focus and think will make them less reactive.

At the same time, when moving them through a chute, keep them moving calmly and steadily. If they stop, they are likely to turn around and want to head back where they came from.

Unlike horses, who will move away from pressure from humans, cattle will turn and face you. Learn where the breakover point is to push them forward or backward.

Don't try to make them go from a large pasture through a small gate by driving them. Funnel it down so the path becomes narrower and they cannot turn away. Or teach them where the gate is. Cattle follow better than they respond to being driven from behind. And don't forget, with their poor depth perception, a gate that we can see is open, might look closed to a cow, and for all she knows you're trying to drive her into the fence for some bizarre reason.

When moving a group of cattle from pasture to pasture, make sure the group is together. Unless the cows are all very familiar with where the gate is and the route everyone else is going, once a lagging cow realizes the rest of the group has left her, she may panic and go through the fence to get to them. And, sometimes, even if she is familiar with the route, the panic at being separated from the herd makes her upset and confused. If a calf gets separated from its mama, it's going to look for the shortest distance back to her, whether that's through, over, or under.

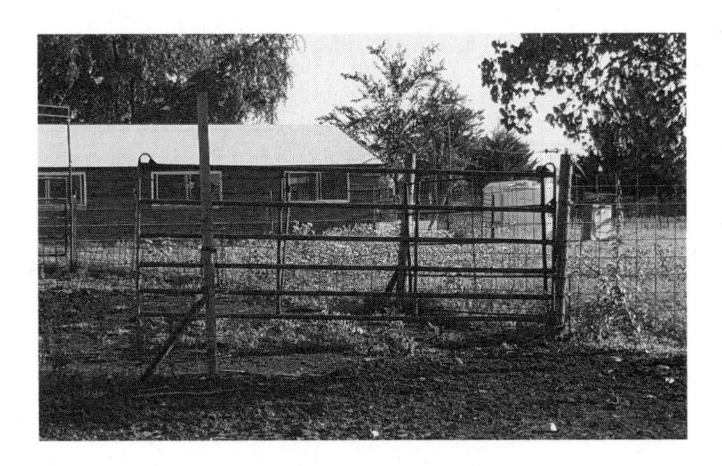

Gate open? Gate closed?

Cattle react negatively in three distinct ways:

Kicking is normally a reaction to a stimulus, such as being startled or pushed. Some cows are more reactive than others and the fact that you have entered their comfort zone can cause them to lash out. They may kick first and see what they kicked later. Cattle that are more reactive can learn to tolerate people approaching and moving behind them, but lashing out will always be a first response if they are startled. Cows are adept at kicking out to the side, much more than straight behind them. And they are fast.

It's impossible to work around cattle and never go behind them. Staying close to the cow can help reduce the force of a kick; the closer you are the less power the kick has, but it can still hurt. A lot.

Your best defense is to watch the cow and how she responds to you. If her head is up, she's looking at you out of the corner of her eye, and her tail is swishing, that's a clear sign that she's not happy.

Horned cattle are amazingly adept at knowing exactly where the tips of those horns are, and using them precisely. In contrast to a reactive kick, when cows point their horns at you, they know exactly what they're doing. They will use their horns to spar with other cattle in the herd for hierarchy or to compete for food or water, and also as a defense if they feel cornered or threatened. Letting cows threaten or jab you with their horns should not be tolerated. Most of the time some negative feedback in the form of a sharp noise, such as clapping hands, stomping feet, or a loud "quit" will give the idea the behavior is not appreciated.

Head butting is a common behavior for calves when they want something. They butt their mother's udder, butt each other in play, and butt to learn to spar and practice finding their place in the herd. It's cute when they are babies; it's definitely not cute when they weigh over a thousand pounds. Bottle-raised calves are especially prone to this behavior, and it should not be tolerated. Again, a sharp word or noise should be sufficient to correct this, and if it is not enough, a sharp swat on the shoulder or nose will clear things up. You aren't being mean. If you've ever watched a herd of cows, you know that they will do way worse to each other. You are not doing them a favor at all by allowing bad behavior, and you are setting up a potentially dangerous situation for other people.

Transporting Cattle

Whether it's bringing them home, taking them to market, taking them to be bred or to the veterinarian, at some point you will need to be able to haul your cattle somewhere.

It is not necessary to own a new, fancy truck and trailer, but you should at least be able to borrow or rent them if you do not own.

Trailers

There are two types of trailers: bumper pull and gooseneck. Bumper pull trailers do exactly that, they hitch to the back of the tow vehicle, either to the bumper itself or, better, to a receiver hitch mounted on the vehicle frame.

A gooseneck trailer is dubbed that because the longer "neck" of the trailer hitch somewhat resembles a goose's long neck.

Gooseneck trailers hitch to a ball in the center of the bed, that is, directly over the rear axle of the tow vehicle. Trucks that are equipped to tow gooseneck trailers have either a permanent hitch ball in the bed of the truck or, more commonly, a hitch ball that can be removed or turned over, so that the ball does not impede using the bed of the truck.

Either trailer is completely serviceable. Bumper pull trailers are often less expensive and smaller. The drawback to bumper pull trailers is that the weight of the trailer rests on the rear of the truck, whether the hitch is on the bumper or a receiver hitch. Because of this, a bumper pull trailer is more prone to swaying while in motion, especially if the load is moving

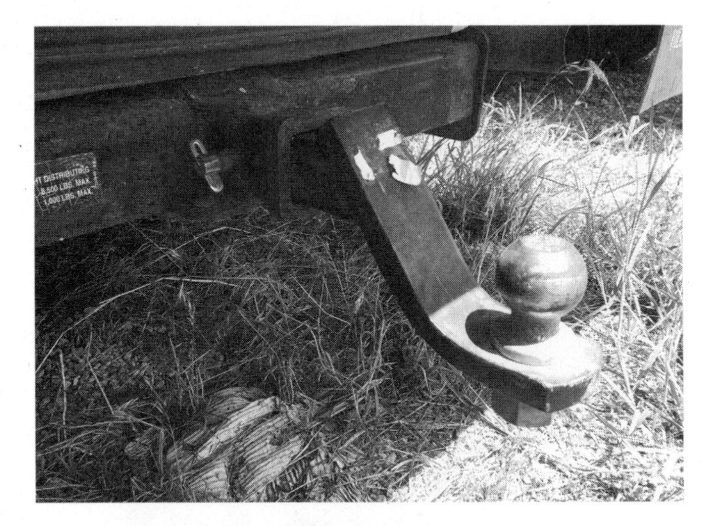

Receiver hitch.

Gooseneck ball.

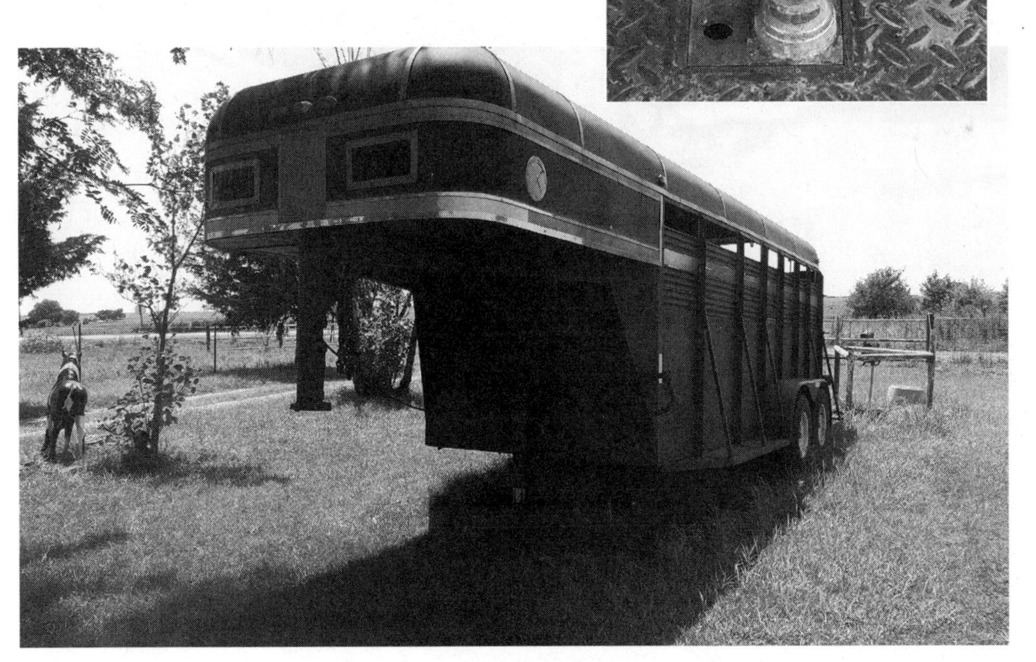

Gooseneck trailer.

around. Under the right (or wrong) conditions, a load can sway so much that it can cause the trailer to wreck. Sway bars can be fitted to the trailer and truck to help reduce this.

Gooseneck trailers have the weight directly over the rear axles, which makes the setup much more stable. They are less prone to swaying and, generally, are easier to pull. The downside is that they do tend to be a little more expensive.

Purchasing a Trailer

A decent trailer of either type can be purchased for a reasonable price, although reasonable can mean different things to different people. Expect to pay a minimum of $2,000–3,000 (US) for a decent gooseneck, about half that for a bumper pull.

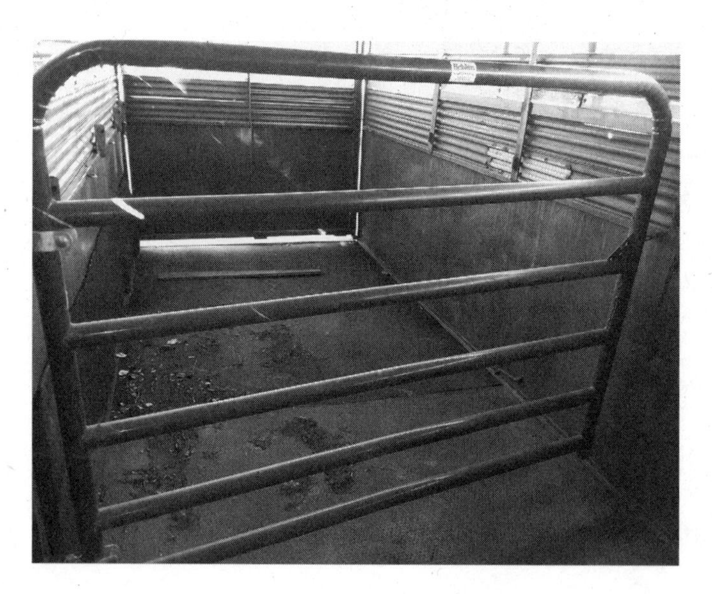

Cut gate.

When looking at the trailer, pay less attention to cosmetic issues. Most trailers that have been farm equipment have sat out in the weather, and the paint may be rusty and faded.

Pay more attention to structural issues such as the floor and rust around the walls. Often farm trailers do not get cleaned out between loads, and the manure and urine left in the trailer can cause the floor to rot and the metal walls to rust. Check the floor to see if it feels solid, and look closely at the joints.

It is extremely helpful for a trailer to have a "cut gate," which is a partition that can be swung across the front half of the trailer, thereby allowing the animals to be separated if necessary.

Wood floors are slippery, and often mats will be added to the trailer for traction. Pull those up if possible, and see what condition the floor is in. If it's pitted and rotten looking, it's dangerous.

Rubber mats provide cushion for the animals' feet and help deaden road noise. If the trailer does not have them, consider adding them.

Check the tires and the spare. Trailer tires do not have to be showroom quality, but look for dry rot cracks and rust around the rims.

Ask if the lights work. Trailer light wiring is notorious for rubbing and breaking just because, and you really do need turn signals and brake lights, or you may discover the hard way how little some motorists pay attention to farm vehicles.

Ask the seller how the trailer has been maintained. Anyone who has taken good care of a trailer is proud of it, and will likely be happy to tell you right up front if the floor has been redone, if they check the grease zerks on the axles, if it's got new tires, etc.

Let me also say that none of these problems are deal-breakers if you can get a really good price on the trailer, but know up front if you need to spend some time and or money to get it to a safe, road-worthy condition.

Make sure you have a jack, safety flares or markers, and a fire extinguisher, and keep them with the tow vehicle. Hopefully, you will never use them, but an emergency is not the time to remember you left them in the garage.

Loading Animals in the Trailer

Hopefully, the place you are picking up your cows from has a chute or some sort of working pen to narrow the cattle down to where they will step on the trailer. A trailer, no matter how nice it is, is a dark scary box to the cows, and it is not in their nature to want to go inside.

Narrowing the path they take can keep them pointed forward instead of turning back, which they tend to want to do. If they turn back several times, your odds of actually getting them on the trailer decrease. They will begin to get worked up, and then you get worked up and frustrated, and it's downhill from there. Once that happens, everybody needs to take a break, go have a sandwich and a glass of water, rethink your setup, and try again. Nothing is gained by trying until someone or something gets hurt.

Getting the cows into a narrow chute or alleyway gives them time to look forward, and if you quietly and calmly provide pressure from behind, once they have a chance to look the trailer over, they will likely go on in.

If cattle have never been loaded on a trailer, the change in flooring will feel very different to them, and they can sense

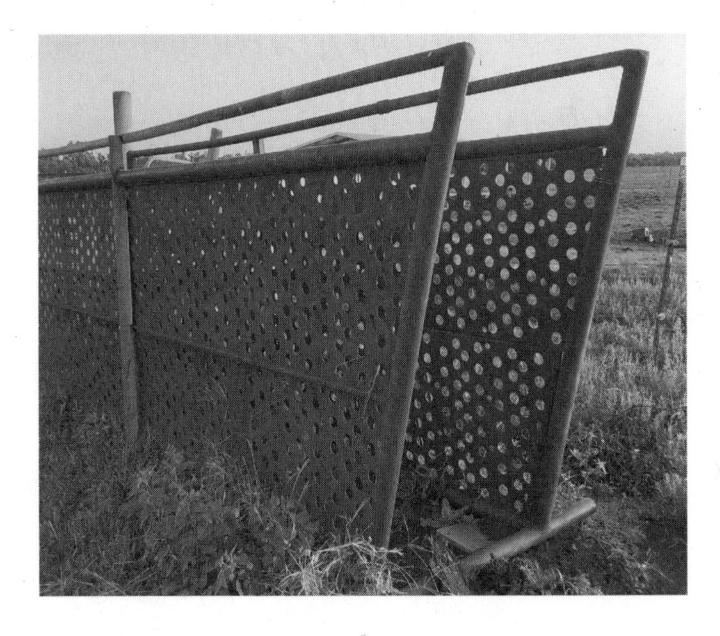

Loading chute.

the trailer isn't as solid as Mother Earth. Give them a second or two to figure it out, continue to apply steady pressure, and they will go in.

It is also helpful to have places where, once the cattle are pointed in the right direction, gates or panels can be shut behind them. They may back up against them, but eventually will figure out that forward is the only place to go.

Once in the trailer, if you are picking up multiple animals, put the heavier animals in front of the cut gate if you have a gooseneck. Distribute the load evenly if it's a bumper pull. And either way, give the animals the minimum space needed to be comfortable. If they move around too much it can cause swaying problems and, honestly, they will be more comfortable in the smaller space.

Trailer driving is a skill like any other. Take it slow and steady, and remember that any move you make with the tow vehicle is compounded in the trailer. Brake slowly, and pay attention to the road ahead of you, way farther ahead than you're used to in a car. Motorists who have never pulled a trailer don't realize that your stopping distance and ability to react safely is at least twice what theirs is. In heavy traffic, don't try to go with the flow. Pick a lane, stick to it whenever possible, and let them go around you. You've got cows! You don't care what they think.

Introducing Cattle to your Farm

When bringing cattle on to your farm, make sure you've checked your fences to make sure they are tight and there are no gaps a crafty bovine can slip through. And if your cattle are young, they can slip through some amazingly tiny spaces.

Especially if you have young animals, they will be a bit disoriented at first and may want to go in search of familiar territory or other familiar animals. If you have a small pen as part of your set up that they can be kept in for the first few days, keep them there, as long as they have shelter and water.

Once they are used to you, and know where feed and water are, it's safe to let them out to explore the bigger pastures.

If you already have cattle and are introducing newcomers, then, once again, putting them in a smaller pen, where they can meet the other cows through the fence and get to know one another, helps a great deal. A single new animal being introduced to an established herd will get picked on, as each animal tries to figure out where the new cow will fit into the herd structure. It's also possible for the new animal to get herded around and run into or through a fence or, if the weather is hot, run around to the point of exhaustion.

Giving them a chance to sniff each other and get all the bluffing and posturing out of the way while the new cow is

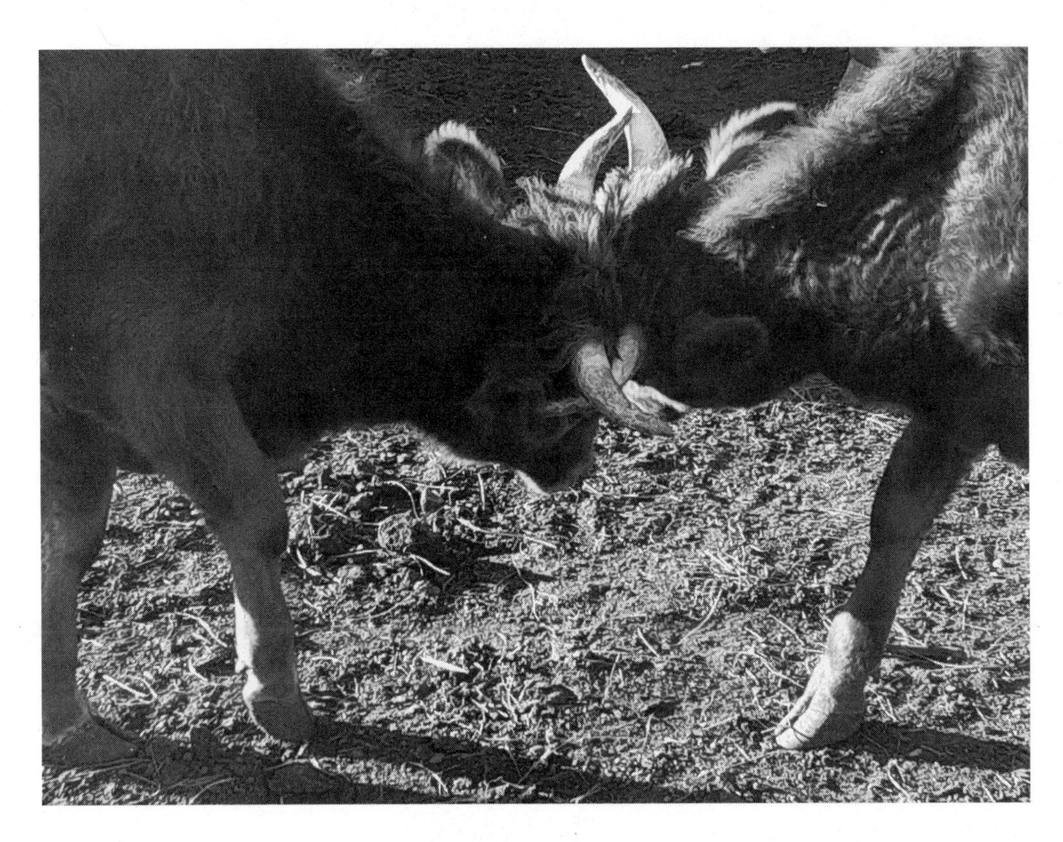

Cattle fighting.

protected by the fence can eliminate a lot of the potential risks of an introduction.

Fencing

Robert Frost was right. Good fences really do make good neighbors. Cattle, given the opportunity, like to roam. A good fence will keep them contained and reduce the chance of you meeting your neighbors in less than desirable circumstances.

Good fencing also reduces your risk of liability, should your cows get out and onto the highway. Laws vary from location to location, but there is a very real chance that if your animals aren't where they are supposed to be, cause a wreck, and injure someone, you might be held liable. Also, anyone can sue anybody in this day and age, and even if you are not found negligent, it's a headache no one needs.

Fencing can be divided into two types: permanent and, well, semi-permanent or moveable. Each has a host of subcategories, but basically permanent fencing revolves around posts anchored in the ground and wire or mesh attached to it.

Of course, any fence can be taken out with enough motivation, but no one digs holes and sets posts in concrete with the notion that they are taking them out next week.

Permanent Fencing

Permanent fencing usually begins with anchor or corner posts, usually wood posts set in concrete. These anchors or corners allow the fencing to be stretched tightly along each line of the fence.

The line posts will usually be T-posts, metal posts that have to be hammered into the ground with a T-post driver. The barbwire, or woven wire, clips to the post, which has nubs evenly spaced so the clips and wire don't slip down easily. This also allows you to make sure the wires are evenly spaced on each post along the whole line, which is very important when you are building fence with a perfectionist! For wooden posts, whether on the corners or on the line, the fence wire is attached with fencing staples.

Barbwire, or barbed wire, is one of the most commonly used cattle fences. It is relatively inexpensive and, even with the barbs, relatively easy to handle compared to large rolls of field fencing.

It works well for cattle, who will tend to want to reach over fence to graze on the other side. The barbs deter them from pushing too hard and eventually stretching and working the wires loose. Barbwire can also be tightened easily, and it's usually highly visible. The majority of the permanent cattle fences, especially in the western states, are barbwire.

Barbwire also has a well-deserved reputation for being nasty. Gloves and long-sleeved shirts are a must when working with it. The barbs like to grab skin, clothing, anything they come in contact with, really, and scratches on your arms and hands are a badge of honor when finished with the fencing job.

There are several thicknesses of barb wire, and it's available in 2- and 4-barb versions.

When allowed to become slack, barbwire can pose a hazard to animals. Lower wires that become loose and lie on the ground can entangle legs. Cattle are normally pretty good about not panicking in that event, but many horse people won't have barbwire within a hundred yards of their farm, just because of the risk of injury.

Fence stays are twisted pieces of wire that rotate down over the strands of barbwire and, when in place, keep the wire from sagging. They work great in areas where it's necessary to have a longer space between T-posts. Generally, T-posts are spaced 10–12 feet apart, but in rocky areas sometimes you can't always put a post exactly where you want it. A stretch much longer than 12 feet will definitely benefit from a fence stay.

Barbwire works great as a perimeter fence around your property, and then fences within can be made with less aggressive or less expensive wire. Barbwire should never be used in an area where animals will be crowded together, such as a working pen or loading chute.

Woven wire, or field fencing is another type of permanent fencing. It usually costs more than barbwire, but it is highly visible and, when tight, very attractive. It is safer to handle because it's not as grabby as barbwire, but the rolls are heavier and difficult, if not impossible, for one person to move.

Woven wire can be used with the same T-posts as barb, and spacing is much the same. One of the drawbacks to woven wire is that it is more difficult to tighten, as the whole span of wire has to be stretched at the same time, rather than individual strands one at a time like barbwire. A mechanical fence stretcher is almost a necessity when putting in field fencing. And, when going back to tighten a field fence, the fence clips will have to be removed to allow the fence to tighten up, whereas barbwire will slide through until it hits the next barb.

Another drawback is that cattle will love to rub on woven wire, and will stretch it until it no longer looks attractive. They can push it until the fence clips pop off and then continue to rub until the whole thing sags. (Yes, I'm speaking from experience.) A strand of hot wire running about shoulder height is a good deterrent.

Woven wire is about as escape proof as fencing can get, though. Calves cannot slip through, and larger cattle won't be able to get their heads through to graze the always-greener stuff on the other side.

Wooden fencing is attractive but often pricey, depending on your location. If you live in a region where wood is plentiful, or even available on your property, this might be more of an option. Wood will ultimately be high maintenance, requiring painting or some sort of protectant, and, ultimately, wood will rot.

Cattle will also enjoy rubbing on a wood fence, so the caveat about a strand of hot wire applies here too.

Corral panels are metal panels with foot loops on the bottom to keep the lowest rail off the ground. They are usually too expensive to be practical for a perimeter fence, although I have seen them used for a much longer stretch than I would ever have wanted to pay for!

Corral panels have a loop on one end and a pin on the other so they can be quickly and easily taken down and moved. They are sturdy and, for the most, part escape proof.

Ornery cattle can bend them, though, either by hitting them or, in the case of one particularly rebellious Pineywoods we have, trying to go underneath. And, once bent up, their usefulness is limited.

Corral panels are best used in areas where the cattle will be crowded together or a sturdy barrier is needed. If you have cattle that are difficult, it's pretty easy to attach a solid piece of plywood to a corral panel to form a visual barrier.

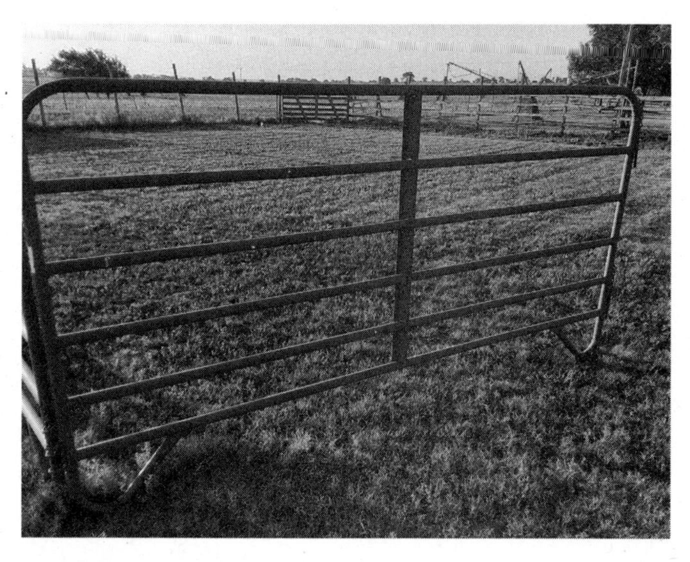

Corral panel.

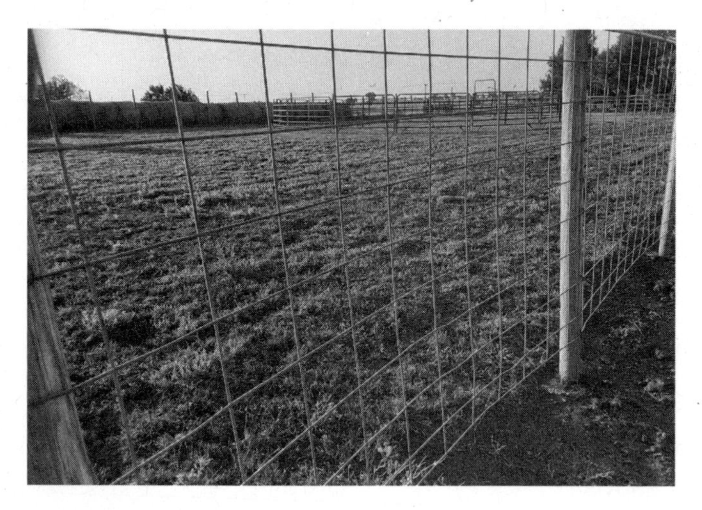

Cattle panel.

Cattle panels are made of galvanized rods that are welded together, forming a panel made of squares. They are generally 16 feet long, and the squares are 4 to 8 inches in size, depending on the type of panel.

These can be wired together to form a temporary fence around a stack of hay bales, for example, or used in conjunction with wood fence to add more support or fill in gaps. They can be attached to wood posts with fencing staples.

Semi-permanent or Moveable Fence

Electrified, or "hot wire," is the quintessential portable fence. Once trained to respect it, cattle will not challenge it, and a single strand can keep a herd confined under most circumstances. An electric fence works by a fence charger pushing a pulsing electric current through a wire. The current is not complete, however, until an animal touches the fence while in contact with the ground. Then the circuit is completed, and the charge is delivered. This is why a bird can rest on a strand of hot wire and not receive a shock; it has not completed the circuit by touching the ground.

Because it will not be challenged as regularly, hot wire does not require to be stretched as tightly, and therefore does not require as substantial a corner set up as barbed or woven.

If your cattle have never been around hot wire, or you aren't certain if they have ever experienced it, take a little time to set up a test run within a larger pasture or paddock. Give them some time to investigate and plenty of room to get away when the inevitable happens. Once they learn, they won't forget.

However, NEVER assume that the hot wire doesn't need to be checked regularly to make sure it's got a charge. Our cattle are very good about not challenging the hot wire... until... it gets grounded out, broken, or the GFCI on the electrical plug has tripped for some reason or another. I don't know whether those cattle can hear, see, or smell that electrical charge going through the fence, but when it's not working, they figure it out pretty quick. Maybe they're just that much smarter than I am.

Electric Fence Equipment

Electric fence wire comes in various gauges—the lower the number, the thicker the wire. Most hot wire available is 14 or 17 gauge, and the thicker 14-gauge wire is usually about twice as expensive as the smaller gauge. The thicker the wire, however, the more surface area it has and the greater the charge it can deliver. Thinner wire always seems to break more easily (as you might expect) and the thinner wire will cause greater injury should an animal become entangled in it.

There are a variety of step-in-the-ground electric fence posts on the market that can make creating internal paddocks for your cattle quite easy. They are light weight, usually made of plastic or poly material, and last several years.

One drawback to standard hot wire is that it is nearly invisible unless you are very close to it. Light colored posts will help give animals an idea that something is there, but when training animals to electric fence, mark it with flagging tape or rag strips tied on the wire so that animals have a chance to see it before blundering into it.

A good electric fence charger is the key to a successful hot wire setup. Fence chargers are either solar, battery powered, or plug in.

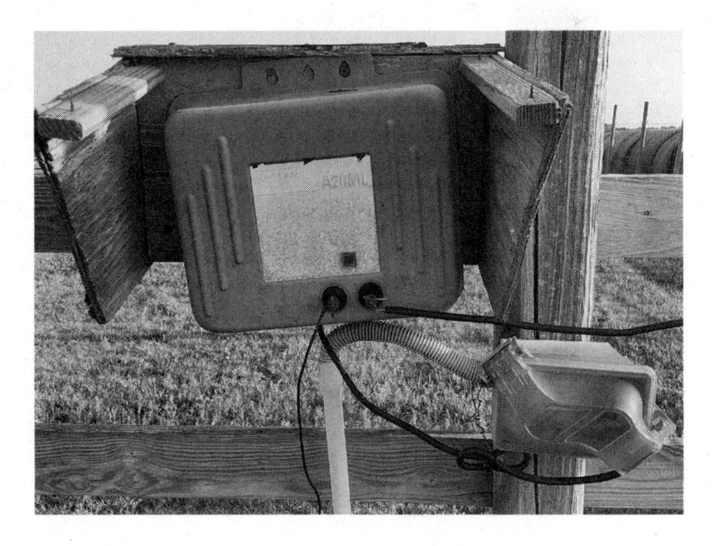

Plug in fence charger.

Plug-in fence chargers will plug into a standard 110 volt electrical outlet. Depending on where this outlet is located, it should have an outdoor, weatherproof covering. Plug-in chargers are usually more powerful and dependable and do not use much electricity, only a few cents per month.

Battery-powered chargers require a separate battery that must be maintained and charged regularly. A low-impedance charger will need a marine deep-cycle battery. Low-impedance refers to the resistance in the charger, not in the fence itself. With less resistance in the charger, more power is delivered to the fence. A low-impedance fence charger is best for stretches of fence through weedy areas.

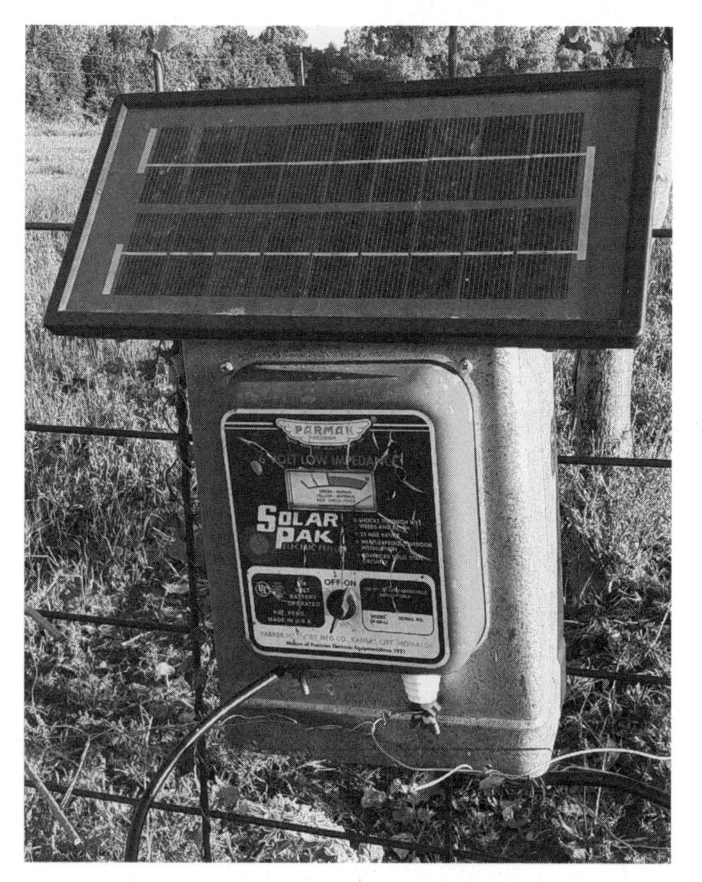

Solar fence charger.

Solar chargers are basically battery-powered models with a solar panel to keep the battery charged. Solar fence chargers are a great option where electrical power is not easily available. They do contain a battery cell that will wear out over time and no longer keep a good charge. Replacement batteries are considerably less expensive than purchasing a whole new charger! Low-impedance solar chargers require more battery power and will generally need a bigger, more expensive solar panel. Solar chargers, once the battery is fully charged, will keep a fence hot even through several days of cloudy weather.

Grounding

One of the key components of a successful electric fence is the grounding system. A good ground rod is necessary as part of the circuit loop of the electric charge. Without the ground rod being in contact with the earth, the circuit will not complete as well. Soil conductivity can affect the quality of the ground system, and in some places with drier soil, multiple ground rods may be needed to get good soil contact. Ground rods should be driven 3–5 feet into the soil whenever possible.

The fence charger will have two output pins, one attached to the line of fence and the other to the ground rod. A good connection to the ground rod is essential.

When soil is dry, it will shrink and pull away from the rod, and the ground rod will not make good contact. If possible, install the ground rod in an area that stays wet naturally. In dry weather, wet the area around your ground rod. This can be done directly with a garden hose or by using a 5-gallon bucket with a small hole in the bottom that will let the water seep out and soak the ground gradually.

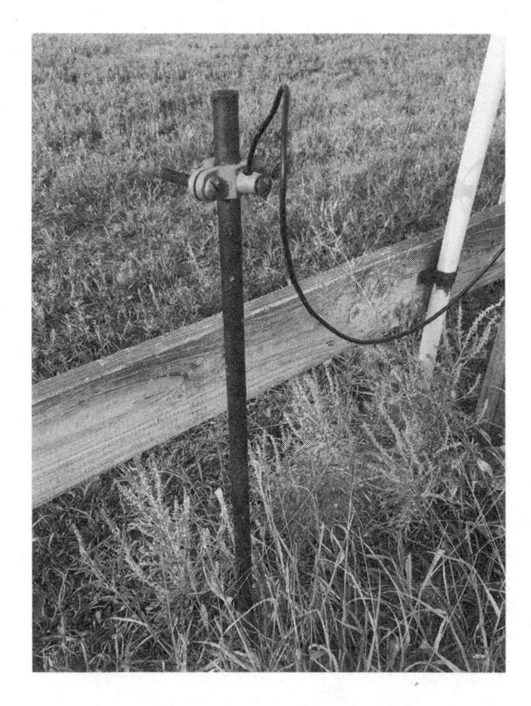

Ground rod.

Troubleshooting Tips

I've gotten my step count in on more than one occasion by walking our hot-wire fence looking for a short. It's always the last place you look (naturally, because why would you keep looking?), and I've developed a few tricks to keep me from having to spend too much time at it.

- Get a good fence tester. The cheaper ones might work fine, but a good one will last years, and one that actually gives you a numerical readout of how much power your fence puts out will help you know if your fence is "OK" or "great"!
- Test your charger output, especially with the solar versions. If your battery is weak and not holding a charge, no amount of fence walking will solve the problem. Check the output by unhooking the fence wire from the charger (turned off first!) and testing the charger without the fence attached. If the output is low, your problem is with the charger or the ground rod. If the tester lights up like Christmas, the problem is in the fence.
- Take a look at your ground rod connections. I once forgot my own advice and spent over an hour walking fence, only to discover that the ground wire end had gotten frayed and brittle over time and was no longer making good contact with the ground rod. Lesson learned.

- A single run of hot wire is pretty easy to check, but if you have multiple stretches of fence and different paddocks running from the same charger, like we do, when you make your connections, make them so you can isolate one stretch of fence at a time from all the others. Then it's just a process of elimination to figure out which stretch of fence has the short.

Corner brace.

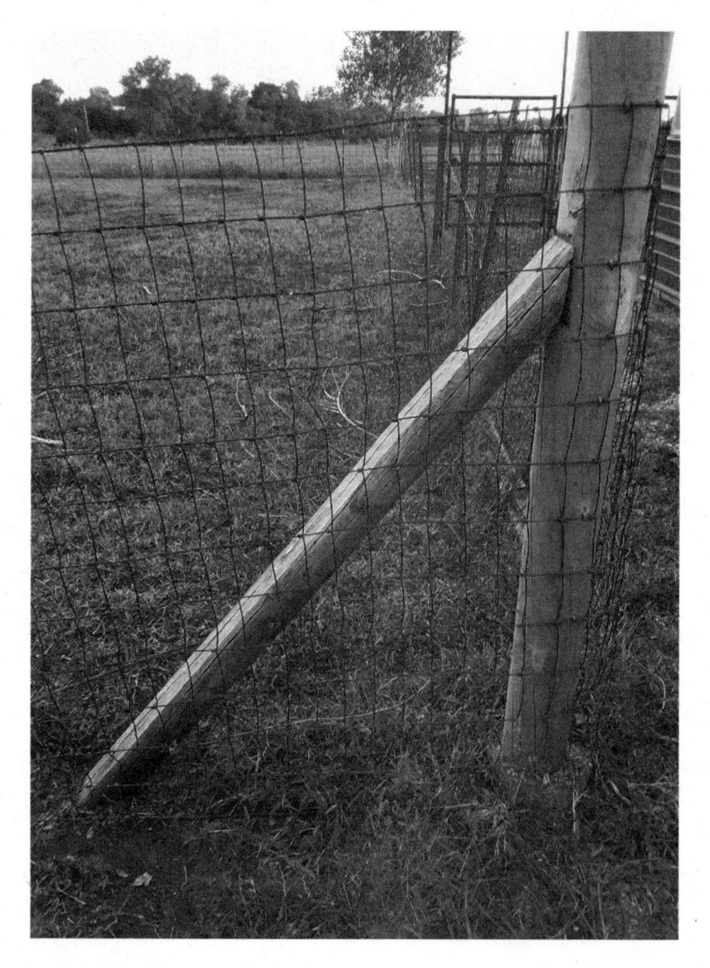

All fencing depends on regular maintenance. Hot wire must be checked regularly, and it's a good idea to always walk the perimeter fence before turning cows in to a pasture for the first time in the grazing season. There is literally no maintenance-proof fence.

Fence Building Tips

- Put the wire on the animal side of the posts. If it's on the outside, as cows rub and push on it, the staples or clips will work loose, and the whole thing can come down.
- Brace the corner posts.
- If you plan to have both cows and a bull at the same time and your plan includes separating them from time to time, then the fence between them should be substantial, and adding a strand of hot wire is a good idea. Bulls have one mission in life, to be with and breed cows. They can be incredibly determined in getting that done, and your fences will suffer.

Facilities and Equipment

Facilities for cattle do not have to be elaborate. Cows are generally easy to keep in that they require very little in the way of barns or equipment. In milder climates, a tree row might be enough to provide shade and shelter from the weather. But in most cases, a three-sided shed will be a good investment and not be too difficult to set up or maintain.

Should you live in an area where winter temperatures can become extreme or predators might be a problem, a barn, or at the least a shed that has a door that can be shut, is probably going to be necessary. That will give you a little more security and peace of mind that your cow isn't out calving in inclement weather or your new calf is not vulnerable to predators. Most cows are very good at taking care of their offspring in most circumstances, but a little extra security can be beneficial.

Bedding such as straw will be helpful if you need to confine your cow for calving or just to make her more comfortable in extreme winter weather.

Of course, the downside to any barn or shed is that it will need to be cleaned out on occasion. A three-sided shed can be scraped out with a tractor loader bucket quite easily and the manure added to a compost pile for later use in the garden.

Handling Facilities

If you have only one halter-broke cow, and that's all you ever plan to have, much more than a good solid place to tie her may not be necessary.

Halter-Breaking

There are lots of stories old timers tell about breaking calves to lead before the county fair by hitching them to the tractor and dragging them until they give in and walk.

It should be no surprise how I feel about that method.

If you want to halter-break a calf to lead, the younger you start the better. Younger animals have not had the length of experience moving around without restraint, so they come to accept it as the norm.

Start with a well-fitting halter and lead rope, and give the calf a chance to smell it and take a look at it. Small calves are easier to restrain, so grab it with your arms around the chest and rump. (You will notice you've run out of hands at this point, so have a helper or be able to get the calf in a corner so the walls help you restrain it.) Wear good leather gloves to protect your hands.

Pull steadily but firmly on the lead rope, and, above all, the minute that calf takes a step forward, *release the pressure on the rope*. A common mistake is to continue pulling, but it is the release of pressure that rewards the calf for stepping forward. One or two steps the first couple of times is good progress.

If your calf is reluctant to move forward, use a short crop or stick to give him a tap on the rump, as you encourage him to step forward. Again, the minute he takes a step, release the pressure on the rope.

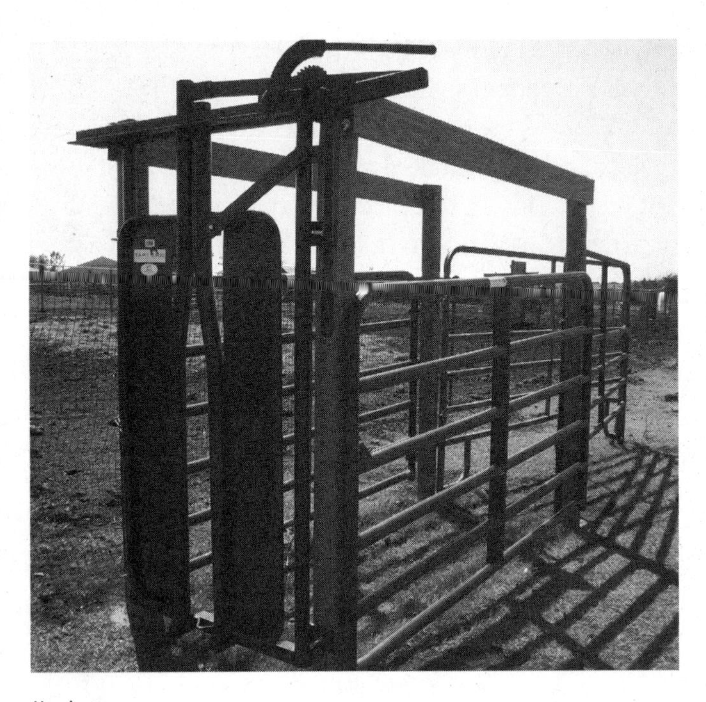

Headgate.

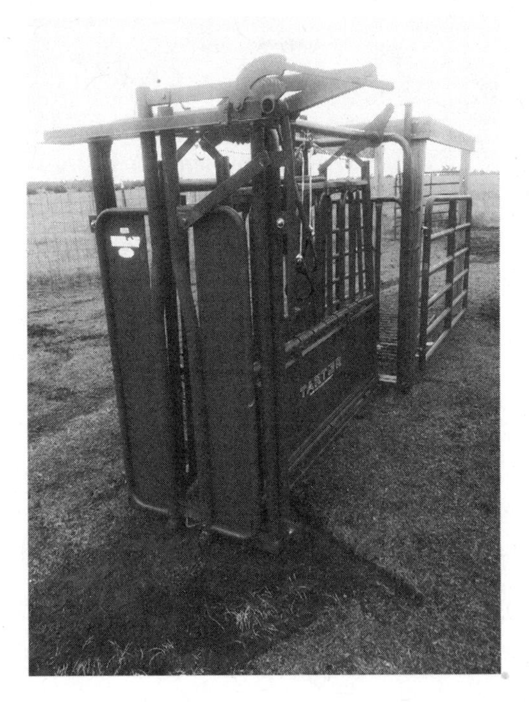

Chute.

Never tie a cow to anything that is not sturdy and anchored. Cows are pretty good about not spooking, but for their safety and yours, any time they are tied it should be securely. Do not tie a cow to a fence rail. Should she pull back, the fence can break. Always tie to an upright, sturdy post for the safest option.

If you have multiple cattle, and no plans to halter-break, some sort of headgate or stanchion can be a lifesaver.

Should you ever need to restrain your cows for vet procedures they need to be held fairly still. A headgate will hold cows solidly and securely and not give them much room to move around, but you still may need additional restraint for safety.

A chute is almost a necessity if you have several cows and plan to do anything such as artificial insemination (AI). Chutes, especially squeeze chutes, reduce the cow's ability to move around, both calming her down and making whatever you need to do safer. It should go without saying that any time you do AI, the last thing you want to do is to have the cow moving around while you are fishing around in her reproductive tract with a stainless steel rod. At best, it will be impossible for you to get it done; at worst, you can do considerable damage to your cow.

A word of advice: if you plan to AI, make sure you do not use a bar or any sort of gate behind your cow to keep her from kicking or backing up. Should she drop down in the chute, your arm can be pinned between the cow and the bar and badly injured. If the cow is squeezed tight enough, she should not be able to kick you during AI. If you are still concerned about getting kicked (I get it, it's not fun at all), a small square bale of straw behind her can protect you and not be hard enough to do as much damage, but have the bale where it can be moved quickly and easily should the need arise.

Also, when asking a veterinarian to work on my animals, I consider it my responsibility to provide as safe a situation as possible for them and to be as prepared as I can be. A good large animal vet is worth their weight in gold these days, and I sure don't want to break mine.

Chutes and Working Pens

Depending on the number of cows you have and your goals, a small working pen and load out chute can be a good investment and save lots of time and frustration. Working pens allow you to narrow the space the cows have, keeping them from running around and you from running after them. Set up correctly, they funnel the cows into the chute or whatever area you need them to be in.

A small catch pen can also be helpful when bringing your cows home for the first time. Having them close can let you get to know them and vice versa, before turning them out on pasture. You can feed them a treat of grain or cow cubes, so both you and the pen will be seen as a source of good things, making them much more willing to come into the pen whenever you need them to.

Try to avoid corners. Cattle will bunch into corners and turn around because they don't quite know where to go. Keep working pens rounded or at least with gradual turns. And, while it can sometimes seem counter intuitive, keeping the space small really does help keep them calm and quiet. (This does not apply to wild range cattle, who will go over, under, and through, but I am certainly hoping you don't start your cattle venture with wild range cattle.)

Hay-Feeding Equipment

We feed large round bales of hay in the winter to our cows. Bale rings are a necessity. If just given a large bale of hay with no ring, cattle will play with the bale, scatter the hay and then use a bunch of it for bedding. If you are a tightwad like me, this is unacceptable. Bale rings keep hay from getting scattered and wasted.

Depending on the area you live in, big round bales may or may not be easily available. They are generally cheaper to purchase than small square bales, and the handling and stacking of small squares becomes less appealing to me as I grow older. I highly recommend large round bales.

Should you have only one cow and don't want to open a big bale and expose hay to the weather, you can set the bale outside the cow area on a pallet and cover it with a tarp. This keeps the hay off the ground but lets you pull off as much as you want to feed at a time.

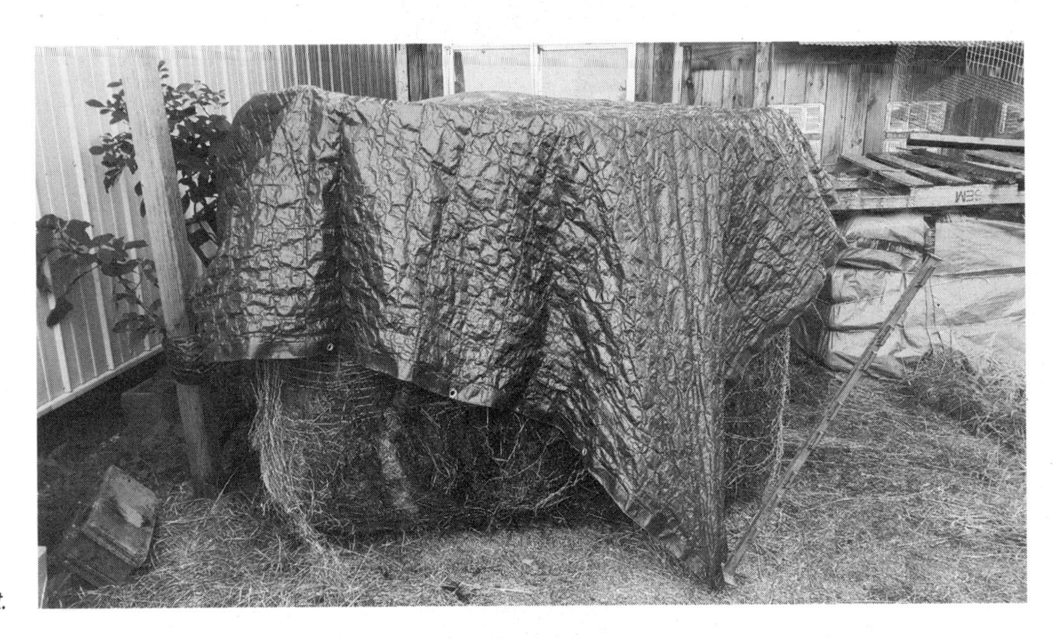

Hay bale on pallet.

Cattle Biology

CHAPTER 4

Forage and Digestion

CATTLE ARE HERBIVORES. Their diet consists strictly of plants. They have no upper incisors, the front teeth used to nip plants; rather they pull plants by grabbing them with their long, dexterous tongue and drawing them between their teeth and the hard palate on the roof of their mouth.

And while we've often heard it said that cattle have "four stomachs," their digestive system consists of four compartments, each with its own unique design and function.

Rumen

The rumen is the largest portion of the digestive system. In a large dairy cow, the rumen volume can range from 25 gallons up to 50 gallons, depending on the size of the cow.

Unlike other organs in the digestive system, the rumen does not secrete enzymes to break down feed but rather functions as a giant fermentation vat.

The slurry of fluid in the rumen contains trillions of microbes, up to 10 *trillion* microbes per milliliter, which do the work of breaking down the cellulose in plant material such as grass and hay and converting them into volatile fatty acids (VFAs), which can be used by the cow for energy.

The wall of the rumen contains thousands of small, finger-like projections called papillae, which help absorb the nutrients from the VFAs.

Technically, as far as the microbes are concerned, the VFAs they produce are waste products. But thankfully, the unique partnership between the cow, the rumen, and the microbes enables the cow to make use of those waste products and obtain high-quality nutrition from otherwise unusable plant material.

The health of both the microbes and the cow depend on the conditions in the rumen remaining in a specific balance. The microbes can tolerate only a small amount of oxygen. Fortunately, the rumen, when healthy and functioning properly, is an anaerobic (without air) environment. The microbes are also intolerant to acidic conditions and begin to suffer if the pH in the rumen drops too far below neutral.

Reticulum

The reticulum is often called the "honeycomb" because of the unique structure and appearance of the wall. Rather than a separate chamber, it is part of the rumen, separated by a fold. Often the whole organ is called the reticulo-rumen. Feed materials freely pass between the rumen and reticulum, with the reticulum collecting smaller particles and moving them to the omasum, while larger particles stay in the rumen to be digested further.

The reticulum also collects any heavier non-feed items the cow might happen to eat. These objects can stay there, but a sharp item like a piece of wire can work its way through the reticulum wall. As the reticulum lies forward in the body cavity, along the diaphragm and close to the heart, these objects can work their way into the heart tissue, causing "hardware disease," a rather benign sounding name for what can be a life-threatening condition.

Omasum

The omasum is the smallest compartment in the cow digestive system, with a volume of about 2 gallons. Its primary function is to absorb water from the digestive tract. Not surprisingly, the material found in this compartment is much drier than the rest of the system.

Abomasum

The abomasum is the "true stomach" of the ruminant and functions much like our own stomach. It secretes digestive enzymes, which further break down food.

In a calf, the rumen is not functioning for about 30 days after birth, even though you will see them imitating mom and sampling what she eats.

When a calf nurses, a groove in the esophagus closes and shunts milk directly into the abomasum, where it can be broken down. Should milk accidentally get into the rumen, it will not digest properly.

This is why it's important for a calf to hold its head in what seems to be an awkward position: the extended neck and jaw allows the esophageal groove to close and do its job.

Rumen and Microbe Health

For optimum health, the rumen needs long-stem forage. Different populations of microbes digest hay and grass than those that digest grains and concentrates. Rapid changes in diet can cause the different populations of microbes to become overwhelmed and can lead to bloat.

Acidosis increases in cattle fed high-concentrate diets. Normal rumen pH can range from 5.7 to 7.6, but at pH lower than 6 the acid intolerant microbes begin to die off quickly, wreaking havoc on the delicate balance in the rumen, and this can cause a life-threatening episode of bloat.

Under normal circumstances, the cow has a built-in rumen buffering system: saliva. A cow can produce 10 to 45 gallons of saliva per day, depending on what she's eating. Saliva has a pH of 8.2. The more long-stem forage the cow has to chew, the more saliva she produces, and the more easily the rumen is buffered. Long-stem forage also provides "scratch factor" in the rumen and stimulates rumen activity.

Another byproduct of rumination is gas, which is normally found on top of the solid and liquid contents of the rumen. As gas builds up, pressure receptors stimulate the esophagus to relax and the cow eructates, or belches.

Contractions in the rumen allow the cow to regurgitate less digested food, and chew it again, further breaking it down. This is what's known as a cow "chewing her cud."

pH

- Neutral pH is 7.0 .
- Water (depending on quality) is neutral pH at 7.0.
- Acidic is anything below neutral. Basic, or alkaline, is above.

Forage Kind and Quality

Poor-quality grass hay is often called "cow hay." Yes, due to the microbial activity in the rumen, cows can make use of poorer quality hay, older hay, or even hay that has gotten wet. But, due to the lower quality and quantity of protein in such hay, they cannot eat enough to meet their minimum protein requirements. Unlike monogastric animals such as horses, once a cow eats enough to fill the rumen, they have to stop eating and allow the microbes to do their job.

The rumen and its residents need a diet with a minimum of 7% protein to function. If the microbes do not get enough protein to function, they won't be able to break down feed as efficiently, and the cow will not thrive.

If your hay is less than 7% protein, which is not uncommon in late-harvest grass hay, you will need to provide with some sort of protein supplement. Adding a flake or two of good-quality alfalfa hay or a scoop of cow cubes can be enough to make everything function optimally.

How Cattle Handle Heat

There are four primary ways cattle can reduce body temperature: convection, conduction, evaporation, and radiation.

Convection happens when air moves across the animal, breaking up the layer of air entrapped by the hair coat. A good breeze or a high-speed fan can increase convective heat loss.

Conduction is from contact with a cooler surface or substance. Cattle standing in ponds are dissipating heat from their lower legs and hooves into the cooler water. This will also happen when they lie on cooler ground, in the shade.

Evaporation happens as moisture dissipates into the air, as from sweat or from panting.

Radiation is the direct transmission of heat from warmer to cooler objects in an environment. Cattle do not lose much heat by radiation on a summer day but they certainly need to be protected from the radiant heat of the sun.

As cattle move from sun into shaded areas, the amount of solar radiation input can be reduced by as much as 50%. Shade is especially important for black-coated cows, as they absorb more solar radiation than light-colored cows. On the other hand, black cows will more effectively radiate heat at night.

Cattle will congregate under shade trees in the summer to get out of the sun. This is good from the point of reducing their radiant heat load, but it also means that they are standing close together and unable to lose as much heat, because everyone is

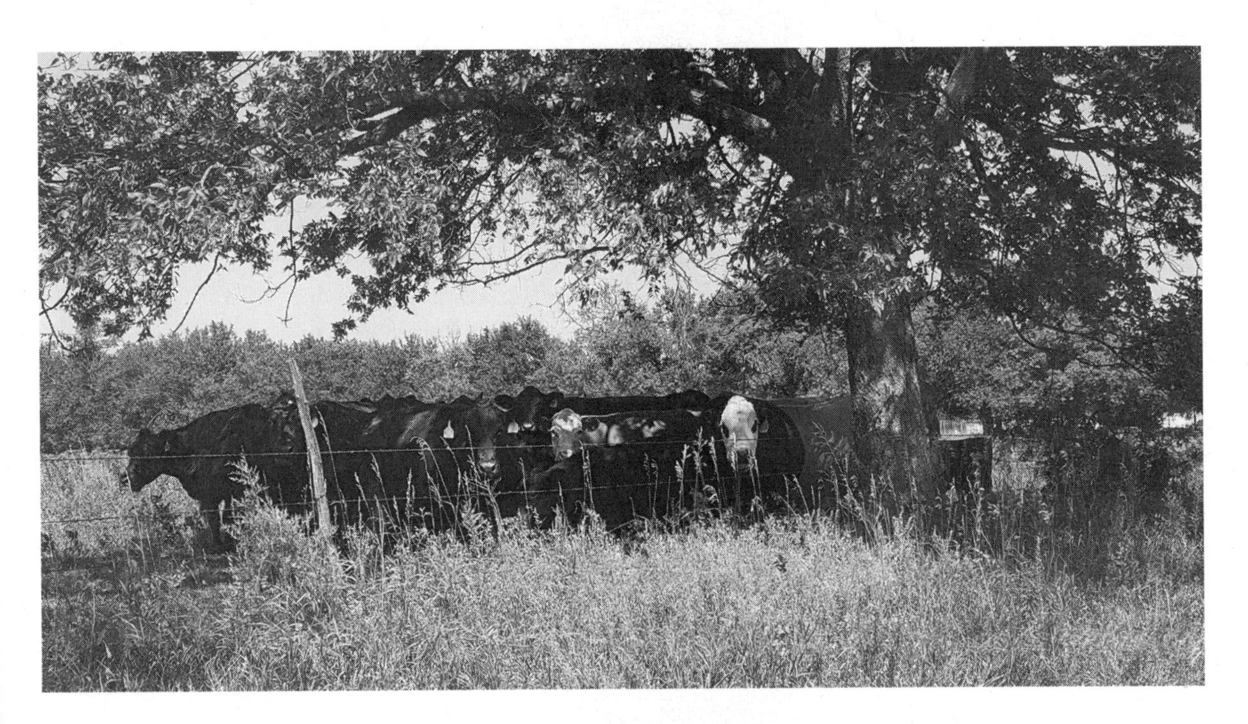

Cows hanging out in the shade.

radiating heat. There should be enough shade available for them to spread out.

It is also important in summer to keep fly control measures in place. Cattle will bunch together to swat each other's flies, and this limits their willingness to spread out.

For conduction, convection, and radiation to be effective, the air temperature must be cooler than the cow's body temperature, normally 101°F (38°C). If the air temperature is higher, then evaporation is the only method of heat loss. And on days when the humidity level is high, evaporation quickly loses its effectiveness.

Cattle can sweat at only about 10% of the capacity that we can. They have minimal sweat glands throughout their hides, and sweat mostly through their noses. Therefore, as it gets warmer, they must pant to exchange heat with the environment. As the environment becomes hotter, they will shift to an open mouth panting. The respiration rate goes down a bit overall, but the energy required to maintain this deeper panting is much greater. A cow that is open mouth panting is stressed and needs to be cooled right away.

Signs of heat stress include

- Panting
- Slobbering
- Uncoordinated movements
- Trembling
- Holding head up to breathe deeply
- Elevated respiratory rate
- Loss of appetite

Should you find a cow in heat stress, move her to shade if she is not already. Cool her by running water over her legs and, if possible, set up a fan to help both with evaporation and pulling heat away from her body. Give her cool water to drink.

Body type and composition affect how much heat a cow's body retains. A smaller-bodied cow, such as a Pineywoods, is much better able to lose heat than a bigger, blockier commercial cow. They can dissipate more heat because it takes less work for the heat to make it to the outside. Something that is thick and square will retain more heat than something thin and narrow.

Lactating animals, young animals, and animals that have respiratory problems are also more prone to heat stress.

Water

Fresh, cool water is essential in the heat of summertime. Not only do cows need water to be able to ruminate, cool water can help reduce their core body temperature, and help them retain less heat.

Water should never be allowed to get green, algae covered, and stale. It's not appetizing to us, and it's not appetizing to cows either. The staler their water is, the less they will drink. (I have seen cows

Heat Index Chart

	80	82	84	86	88	90	92	94	96	98	100	102	104	106	108	110
40	80	81	83	85	88	91	94	97	101	105	109	114	119	124	130	136
45	80	82	84	87	89	93	96	100	104	109	114	119	124	130	137	
50	81	83	85	88	91	95	99	103	108	113	118	124	131	137		
55	81	84	86	98	93	97	101	106	112	117	124	130	137			
60	82	84	88	91	95	100	105	110	116	123	129	137				
65	82	85	89	93	98	103	108	114	121	128	136					
70	83	86	90	95	100	105	112	119	126	134						
75	84	88	92	97	103	109	116	124	132							
80	84	89	94	100	106	113	121	129								
85	85	90	96	102	110	117	126	135								
90	86	91	98	105	113	122	131									
95	86	93	100	108	117	127										
100	87	95	103	112	121	132										

Vertical Axis = Temperature in °F
Horizontal Axis = Relative Humidity in %

	Caution
	Extreme Caution
	Danger
	Extreme Danger

drink out of highly questionable puddles after a rainstorm, yes. But that doesn't mean those should be considered their primary water source.)

As a rule of thumb, cattle will drink 1 gallon per 100 lbs. of body weight in cool weather and 2 gallons per 100 during hot; and lactating cattle will need even more.

Cold Weather

Cattle have a bit of an advantage in the winter. Rumen activity and the fermentation of forage can raise their body temperature a degree or two. Having good hay available so they have plenty to eat and ruminate with will help them tolerate colder temperatures.

Wind and wet weather produce more cold stress than just the ambient temperature does. We've all felt the impact of wind on a cold morning, and if rain or mud is present, the impact is greater.

Cattle need more energy during cold weather, even though their protein requirements remain the same. Cattle do not benefit by having grain added to their diet as much as they benefit from extra forage.

The amount of cold that cattle can tolerate is dependent on weather conditions. A cow with a heavy, dry winter coat can withstand temperatures well below freezing, but if the coat is wet, then even at a temperature of 45–50°F (7–10°C) they will have to spend a lot more energy maintaining their body temperature.

Snow is usually preferable to rain or sleet. If the coat is wet, it provides very little insulation. A dry, thick, coat provides little pockets of air between the hairs, and this provides additional insulation. Wet, matted hair loses this extra warmth. While you might think that a cow with a thick layer of snow on its back is suffering, the animal cannot be losing much body heat if snow won't melt on its back.

Going into winter with cattle in good body condition is also helpful. Not only will the extra flesh provide insulation and heat retention, they will have an extra reserve to draw on during snaps of bad

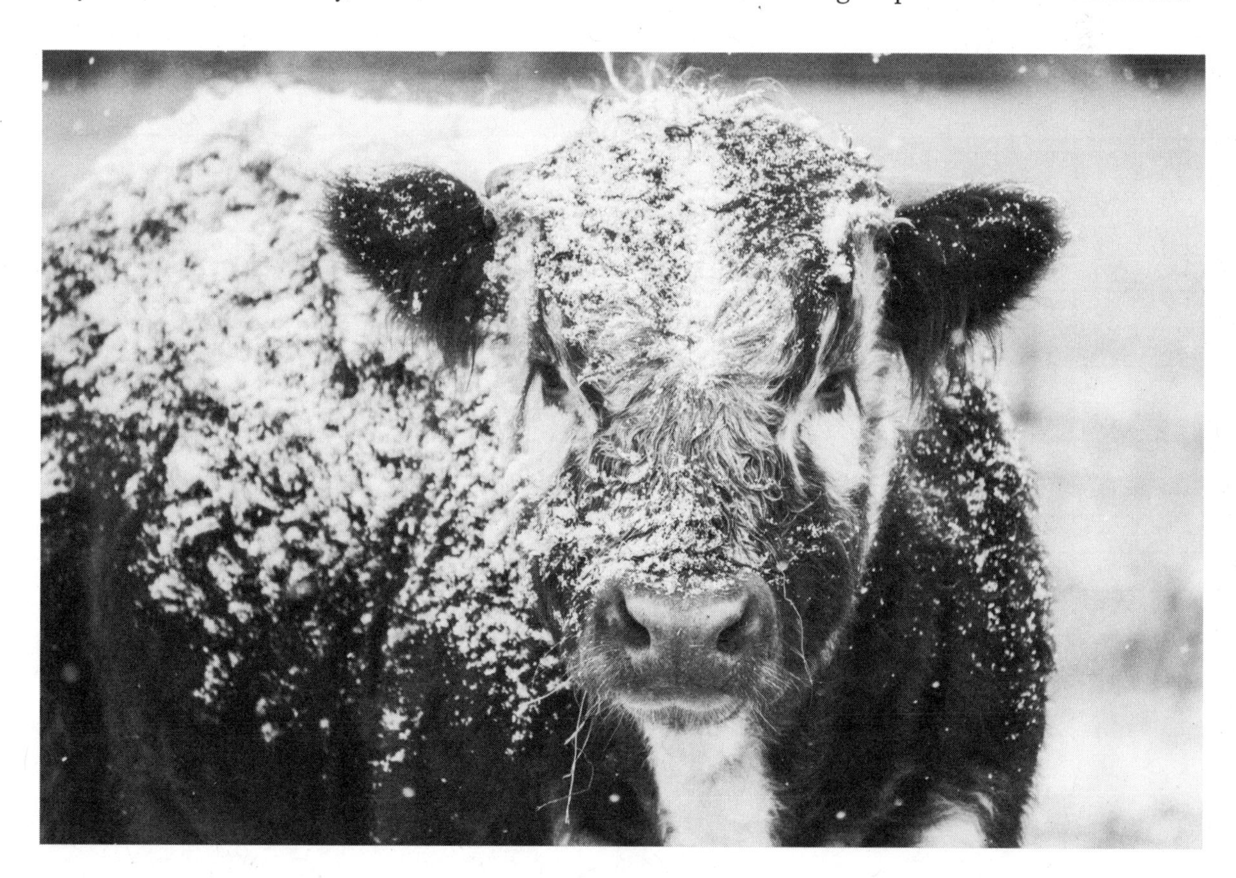

A well-conditioned steer with snow on his back.
Credit: Emily Nyman

weather. It's not uncommon for cattle to lose a bit of condition in the winter. But if they are able to go into cold weather in ideal body condition, they will likely come out in spring in better shape than they would otherwise, and cows that will calve in the spring need to be in good condition to avoid calving problems.

Water

Water is even more critical in the winter than in the summer. Warmer temperatures will encourage cattle to drink more, but in the winter if water intake is reduced too much, rumen activity can be reduced. Providing a salt or mineral block can help stimulate them to drink.

Cattle won't eat without water. Water tanks should be clear of ice, and don't expect cattle to eat snow to get water. Even if they can ingest enough snow to meet their needs, the majority of their time will be spent eating snow, not hay, and the energy required to metabolize the snow will reduce their ability to gain weight or keep their body condition up.

Wind Chill Chart

Calm	40	35	30	25	20	15	10	5	0	-5	-10	-15	-20	-25	-30	-35	-40
5	36	31	25	19	13	7	1	-5	-11	-16	-22	-28	-34	-40	-46	-52	-57
10	34	27	21	15	9	3	-4	-10	-16	-22	-28	-35	-41	-47	-53	-59	-66
15	32	25	19	13	6	0	-7	-13	-19	-26	-32	-39	-45	-51	-58	-64	-71
20	30	24	17	11	4	-2	-9	-15	-22	-29	-35	-42	-48	-55	-61	-68	-74
25	29	23	16	9	3	-4	-11	-17	-24	-31	-37	-44	-51	-58	-64	-71	-78
30	28	22	15	8	1	-5	-12	-19	-26	-33	-39	-46	-53	-60	-67	-73	-80
35	28	21	14	7	0	-7	-14	-21	-27	-34	-41	-48	-55	-62	-69	-76	-82
40	27	20	13	9	-1	-8	-15	-22	-29	-36	-43	-50	-57	-64	-71	-78	-84
45	26	19	12	5	-2	-9	-16	-23	-30	-37	-44	-51	-58	-65	-72	-79	-86
50	26	19	12	4	-3	-10	-17	-24	-31	-38	-45	-52	-60	-67	-74	-81	-88
55	25	18	11	4	-3	-11	-18	-25	-32	-39	-46	-54	-61	-68	-75	-82	-89
60	25	17	10	3	-4	-11	-19	-26	-33	-40	-48	-55	-62	-69	-76	-84	-91

Vertical Axis = Wind Speed in MPH
Horizontal Axis = Temperature in °F

Frostbit Times	
	30 Minutes
	10 Minutes
	5 Minutes

Nutrition and Feeding

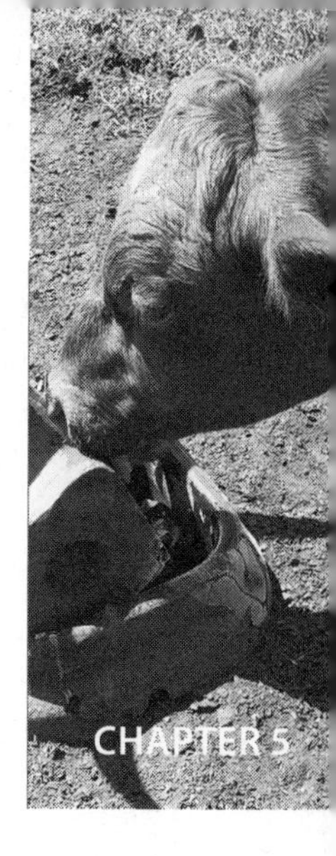

Major Nutrients

THERE ARE FIVE MAJOR CATEGORIES of nutrients: energy, protein, vitamins, minerals, and water. If any one of those is not present in sufficient quantities, the entire metabolic process will not function. A nutrient that is absent or not found in sufficient quantity is called a limiting nutrient.

Energy

Energy in livestock diets is commonly defined in Mcals, or mega calories. One Mcal equals one million calories. Energy is the most important nutrient for any animal, and generally the first limiting nutrient. If energy needs are not met, none of the other essential functions can happen, or happen efficiently. Energy fuels every metabolic process in the body: growth, reproduction, milk production, digestion, and helping to regulate body temperature. Energy needs change depending on what stage of life the animal is in.

In cattle, energy is produced by the metabolism of carbohydrates, such as starches or cellulose, and fat. For the ruminant, fat is a poor source of energy, as rumen microbes are not very good at breaking down fat. Starches are found in grains such as corn or soybeans. Starches can be broken down in the rumen, as discussed in the previous chapter, but too much starch can lead to rumen acidosis.

The best source of energy for a ruminant is good, long-stem forage, in the form of pasture or good hay. The majority of a cow's nutritional needs can be met by either of those two types of cellulose.

Rumen microbes break down cellulose into energy, which feeds the cow and also feeds the microbes so they can continue their work.

When cattle eat, they can consume only so much forage before they get full and have to stop eating to ruminate, allowing what they have eaten to be processed. When the rumen contents have been processed and the rumen is empty, the cow will get up and eat again. This is why good-quality, properly managed pasture is one of the best feeds for cattle. The more they can fill their rumen with highly nutritious forage, the more the microbes have to work with.

Protein

Protein is the second major nutrient cattle need. While the rumen microbes will break down cellulose into VFAs (the building blocks of protein), the ruminant also needs to consume a certain level of protein in the diet for the microbes to thrive. Protein and energy are closely linked when talking about cattle diets.

If all a cow has to eat is stemmy, poor-quality hay, low in protein, she may not be able to eat enough to meet her protein requirements. When her rumen gets full and she has to stop eating to digest, she won't have taken in enough protein and energy to meet her needs.

Cattle on low-quality hay or pasture may need a protein supplement in their diet. If more is fed than necessary, it will be converted to energy or excreted.

Vitamins

Vitamins are essential for many metabolic processes in cattle, and their lack can cause serious health problems.

Fortunately, most of them are easily available in good forage or synthesized in the rumen.

Vitamin A is found naturally and in abundance in good pasture grasses. Cattle can store Vitamin A in their liver, and as grass quality declines through the growing season, they can mobilize stored Vitamin A to make up deficiencies.

Unfortunately, Vitamin A is rapidly destroyed in hay during storage, therefore the most likely time to experience a Vitamin A deficiency is in winter when feeding stored hay.

Vitamin D is synthesized in the cow's own body, with exposure to sunlight.

Vitamin E is also found in sufficient quantities in forages and grains but is killed by heat processing of grains. Vitamin E helps with storage and absorption of Vitamin A, and where a deficiency of Vitamin E occurs, Vitamin A deficiency is also likely.

Vitamin K is synthesized in the rumen under most feeding conditions, and deficiency is rarely a problem. However, moldy sweet clover hay can trigger symptoms of a Vitamin K deficiency by producing a compound called dicoumarol, which interferes with normal Vitamin K activity.

All of the B vitamins are synthesized in the rumen by microorganisms in sufficient quantity that in normal conditions supplementation is not necessary.

Minerals

Minerals are classified as either macrominerals, which are required in relatively large amounts in the diet, or microminerals, which are required but in much smaller doses.

Probably two of the most important macrominerals are calcium (Ca) and phosphorous (P). Calcium and phosphorous are important for the development of bones and teeth but are also critical for certain cellular functions. Forages are usually good sources of calcium. Legumes are higher in calcium than grasses, and grains are usually low in calcium. Because of this, cattle on a high-grain diet may need additional calcium.

There is a whole list of microminerals, and people have literally gotten PhDs in how each of them functions in the cow and how they relate to one another. Most of them are found in forages, but the content of each one can vary widely from one geographic region to another. In the US, your local extension service will have all that info and can tell you if certain minerals are lacking in forages in your area and therefore need special supplementation. In Canada, the Ontario Ministry of Agriculture, Food, and Rural Affairs offers good research materials, and other Canadian provinces will each offer their own localized services.

You may also find that minerals are found in excess, in either or both the soil (and therefore the forage) and the well water. In excess, certain minerals can compete with one another and inhibit how those minerals function. In general, one of the simplest remedial steps to take is to provide cattle with a trace mineral salt block. These are available at any farm

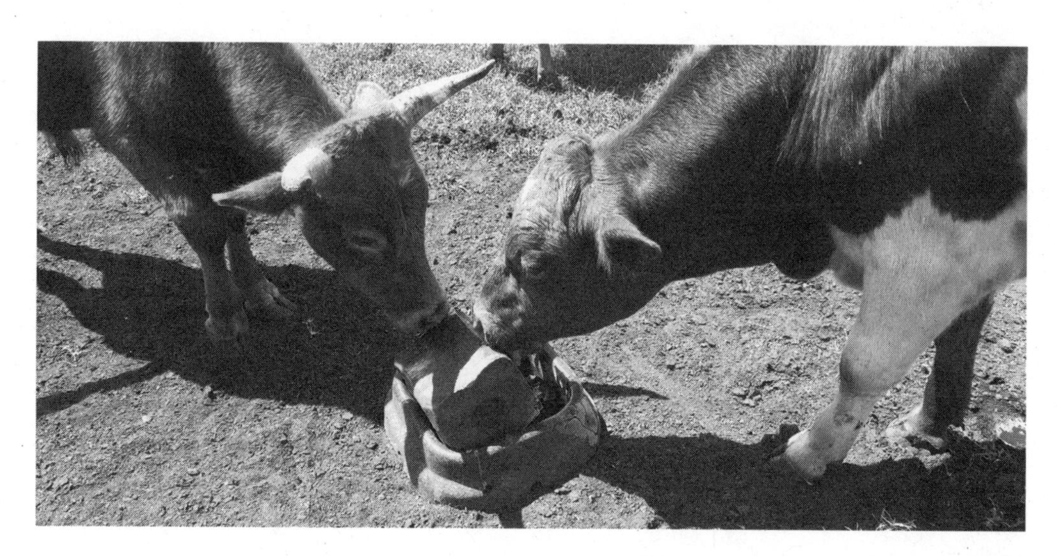

Cattle enjoy a new salt block.

supply store, and the salt has the added benefit of stimulating the cow to drink water. This brings us to our last major nutrient: water.

Water

We don't often think of water as a nutrient, but without it nothing can function, neither on the cellular level nor on a whole-system level. Fresh clean water is essential. A lactating cow in the summer can drink up to 20 gallons of water *per day*. Warm weather will usually ensure that cattle are motivated to drink. In the winter, providing salt to stimulate thirst will also ensure they drink an adequate amount.

Concentrates

Concentrates are the cereal portion of a grain, such as corn or wheat. They are higher in energy and protein and much more easily digestible than forage. Even though the bovine digestive system is designed to thrive on forage, concentrates and grains do have a place in the diet.

Calf starter feed can help a bottle calf or weanling make the transition from milk to a forage diet without losing too much weight. Grains can help a feeder animal finish at a higher weight, and with more marbling.

Grains can also help make up nutritional deficiencies in lower protein grass hay, and provide a boost of energy and protein to keep cattle from losing condition in winter, or during lactation.

Also, cows that are on a higher level of production, such as dairy cows, will need concentrates to be able to sustain their level of production without losing too much condition.

Be aware that problems can occur when concentrates are added to the diet too quickly, or in too large a proportion of the diet, or are ground so finely that they irritate the rumen.

Concentrates should be added in slowly, to give the rumen time to adapt. Start out at 1% of the animal's body weight daily, and increase over a 2–3 week period.

Cattle entering a feedlot have to transition from pasture to grain based diets quickly, so they will be given additives to help prevent rumen acidosis, and will be slaughtered before long term problems begin to show up. Feedlots will pay more for "preconditioned" calves that have already been started on concentrates.

Cattle will grow slower on a forage only diet, and may experience seasonal dips in performance if raised solely on pasture.

Choosing Quality Hay

At some point, the odds are you will need to feed hay to your cattle. Choosing good-quality hay to feed in the winter can make the difference between cows

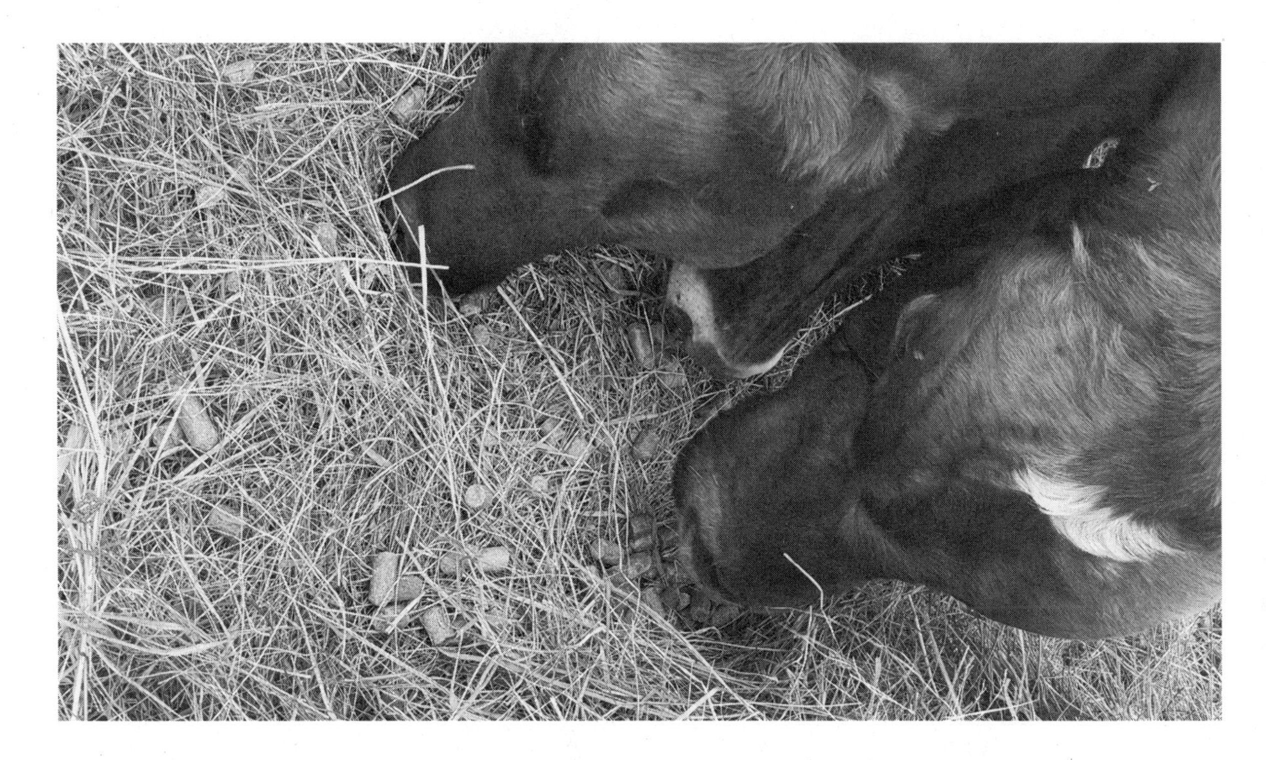

Pineywoods enjoying cubes.

maintaining condition and production and going into spring with the reserves needed to calve or give milk, and starting out already behind.

Hays are divided into two subgroups: legumes and grasses.

Grass hay is just that, grass that has been harvested, baled, and stored until needed to feed. Grass hay is divided further into warm-season grass and cool-season grass. As you might expect from the names, warm-season grasses grow once the soil temperature gets above 60–65°F (15–18°C) and are most active in the warmest months of the year. Cool-season grasses, conversely, are most active in the spring and fall and will go dormant in the hot part of the year.

Grass hay is at its highest nutrition value right before it "heads out" (begins producing seed). This is the ideal time to harvest hay, but it's a pretty short window, and often hay has gone to seed before it can be harvested. This does not mean it's bad hay; it just means it is not at its peak protein level. And remember, hay that is harvested and baled at that perfect stage will likely command a premium price as well.

There are many types of grasses throughout North America that can be cut and baled.

Grasses and Legumes

Cool-Season Grasses
Orchardgrass
Kentucky Bluegrass
Tall Fescue
Perennial Ryegrass
Brome grass
Reed Canarygrass
Timothy
Warm-Season Grasses
Switchgrass
Big Bluestem
Indian Grass
Little Bluestem
Eastern Gammagrass
Legumes
Alfalfa
Red Clover
White Clover
Birdsfoot Trefoil
Alsike Clover

Legumes are plants that have nitrogen-fixing nodes on their roots, which contain bacteria that are able to take nitrogen from the atmosphere, convert it to ammonium, and "fix" that nitrogen in the soil. Because of that nitrogen-fixing ability, legume hay is higher in protein than grass hay. Good alfalfa hay, harvested at the pre-bloom stage, can have 18% protein or higher. Other legumes include clover, lespedeza, and birds-foot trefoil, but alfalfa is the most common legume hay crop. Because of its unique qualities, alfalfa can be harvested multiple times a year, although the total yield per acre will decrease. Alfalfa is also a rather water-intensive hay, and many premium alfalfa fields are irrigated.

If you are choosing alfalfa hay, make sure it is free of blister beetles, an insect most often found in first-cutting alfalfa. These bugs contain a toxin that remains even after they die, which can cause blisters and lesions in the digestive tract of cattle and can be lethal to horses. Studies show that the beetles are attracted to the pollen in the alfalfa blooms, hence the importance of cutting alfalfa before it blooms.

Good grass hay should be bright green in color. Hay that is brown has been harvested later or gotten wet in the harvest process. Hay that is brown can still be fine as forage for cattle, but the cows should be monitored to make sure it is meeting their nutritional needs and that they are holding condition well.

Hay that has gotten wet during the baling process will also not be quite as nutritious but can also be fine to feed if properly raked and allowed to dry. It should not cost as much as hay harvested under prime conditions.

If hay has not cured properly before baling, it can mold within the bale. Cattle can tolerate a little mold in their hay, but too much mold can cause problems. And send you looking for a new hay supplier. A good hay supplier will not knowingly sell you an inferior product.

If hay is harvested later in its growing season, it can also become stemmier. This means the leaf-to-stem ratio (the blades of grass are called leaves) is low; the more leaves and fewer stems, the better the quality of the hay. Again, cattle have little problem chewing up and eating coarser, stemmy hay, but it should be priced accordingly.

When evaluating hay, grab a handful of it and see if it bends or breaks. Hay with good moisture content should mostly bend. Dried, poorer-quality hay will break when twisted. Hay should also smell fresh. Hay that smells musty or moldy should be avoided. A little dust in hay isn't a deal breaker, but a lot of mold, which appears as whitish gray spots in the hay, should be. Bales of hay that are kept outside on the ground will more than likely have mold on the surface that touches the ground, but the mold should not be found throughout the bale.

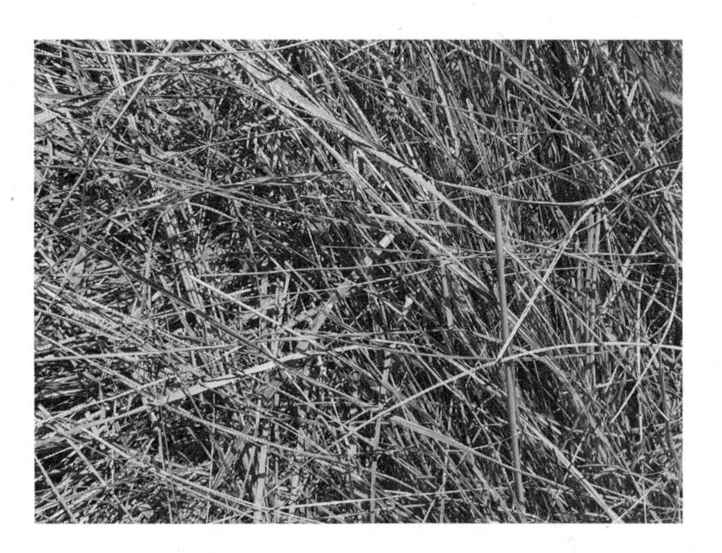

Good-quality hay.

Body Condition

Body condition scores are a quick and easy way to make sure your animals are fit and healthy. This system involves giving each animal a numeric score, based on several visible factors. It's a good idea to evaluate your animals on a quarterly basis, especially going into and coming out of winter and before calving and after weaning. You should be looking at your cows regularly, but it's best to go out and take a look at them with the score chart in hand, or at the very least be intentional in your evaluation. Changes happen over time—when seeing your cows regularly, you become accustomed to how they look in the moment, and changes can sneak up on you. A good intentional evaluation can make sure a change does not become too drastic.

If a cow falls below the ideal range, it's time to evaluate your feeding program, think about weaning her calf, or consider of a number of other factors. She may need concentrates added to her diet, a better-quality hay, or even just more or better pasture. Cows that are too thin will be less likely to rebreed and carry a calf, and being too thin causes systemic stress that can lead to a host of other problems.

If she's above ideal, it's also time to evaluate your feeding program but from the opposite angle. Cows that are too fat are prone to calving problems and can also be difficult to get pregnant. And, at the least, they are hitting you in the wallet harder than necessary.

Because dairy cattle spend their energy making milk rather than meat, even a well-conditioned dairy cow will likely have hip bones more visible than expected on a beef animal. The general points of observation are still similar, however.

Another good measure of a cow's overall health is her hair coat. Hair needs protein, minerals, and vitamins to be shiny and healthy. A deficiency in any one of those categories will often show in the hair coat.

An undernourished cow will have a hair coat that is rough and wiry, and she may not shed her winter hair when the weather turns warm. Or her hair coat may come out in patches, leaving longer hair in some places, and patches may be bald in extreme cases. The hair may also

Guide to Body Condition Scoring in Cattle

	BCS	Spine	Ribs	Hooks/Pins	Tailhead	Brisket	Muscling
Thin	1	Visible	Visible	Visible	No fat	No fat	None/atrophy
	2	Visible	Visible	Visible	No fat	No fat	None/atrophy
Borderline	3	Visible	Visible	Visible	No fat	No fat	None
	4	Slightly visible	Foreribs visible	Visible	No fat	No fat	Full
Optimum Condition	5	Not visible	1 or 2 may be visible	Visible	No fat	No fat	Full
	6	Not visible	Not Visible	Visible	Some fat	Some fat	Full
Over-Conditioned	7	Not visible	Not visible	Slightly visible	Some fat	Fat	Full
	8	Not visible	Not visible	Not visible	Abundant fat	Abundant fat	Full
	9	Not visible	Not visible	Not visible	Extremely fat	Extremely fat	Full

Adapted from Herd & Sprott, 1986; BCS = Body condition score
CREDIT: DR JUSTIN WAGGONER, KANSAS STATE UNIVERSITY

become discolored, and faded. Hair on a black cow may have a rusty tone to it, and yellow hair may bleach to nearly white.

Cattle that have a heavy parasite load may show many of those symptoms, as well as cattle that are fighting some disease or infection. In both of those conditions, nutrients that should go to maintaining the animal go into fighting the parasite or illness.

Most diet recommendations are based on the animal's weight, but very few people have access to a large-animal scale. Each breed has a range that the majority of animals fall into. If your cows fall into the ideal range of body condition, you can get a rough idea of your cows' weight. For example, if a cow is from a breed that should weigh between 800 and 1,000 lbs. and that cow is in ideal condition, then it should weigh pretty close to the 900-lb. mark. There are a whole lot of factors that can come into play, but this can give you a ballpark number to start with.

Determining Supplemental Feed Needs

First, determine the nutritional content of the hay you plan to feed. (Your local extension agent can help you with this.) A hay analysis involves taking a core sample from several of the hay bales, mixing the sample in a plastic bag, and submitting it to a lab for analysis. Many factors can affect the quality of the hay: the forage species, when it was harvested, how much it has weathered, etc. Hay can even vary from one part of a field to another. That is why it is important to get a variety of samples.

Labs typically offer two types of forage analysis, near infrared reflectance spectroscopy (NIR) or wet chemistry. The wet chemistry is more accurate, but is more expensive and takes longer and is generally better used for grains. The NIR will provide all the information necessary much more quickly and economically.

You will receive a printout from the lab with a whole bunch of numbers, but the main ones you will be interested in are dry matter, crude protein, and energy.

Dry matter (DM) is everything that is in the feed, except water. There can be a great deal of variation in the moisture content of forages, so keeping the water out of the equation allows us to more accurately evaluate the nutrient content of the hay. It is usually expressed as a percentage.

Crude protein (CP) is the measure of nitrogen in the diet. Nitrogen is integral to amino acids, which are the building blocks of protein. Depending on the lab, there may be lots of other protein types and percentages, but CP will work for estimating what our supplement needs are.

Energy is listed as the total digestible nutrients (TDN) of the feed. TDN is a very commonly used measure of energy;

Analysis of a Late-Harvest Large Round Prairie Hay Bale

	Dry Basis	As Received	
Moisture		10.04	%
Dry Matter		89.96	%
Protein, Crude	5.16	4.64	%
ADF-Acid Detergent Fiber	42.04	37.82	%
NEL: Net Energy-Lactation	0.49	0.44	Mcal/lb
NEG: Net Energy-Gain	0.19	0.17	Mcal/lb
NEM: Net Energy-Maintenance	0.52	0.47	Mcal/lb
TDN: Total Digestible Nutrients	49.29	44.34	%
Calcium	0.63	0.57	%
Phosphorus	0.06	0.05	%

Analysis of Good Alfalfa Hay

	Dry Basis	As Received	
Moisture		15.73	%
Dry Matter		84.27	%
Protein, Crude	23.32	19.65	%
ADF-Acid Detergent Fiber	25.42	21.42	%
NEL: Net Energy-Lactation	0.73	0.62	Mcal/lb
NEG: Net Energy-Gain	0.47	0.40	Mcal/lb
NEM: Net Energy-Maintenance	0.80	0.67	Mcal/lb
TDN: Total Digestible Nutrients	70.72	59.59	%
Calcium	1.63	1.37	%
Phosphorus	0.31	0.26	%

it is also known to overestimate the energy value of roughages. And energy is often a more limiting nutrient than protein.

The amount of nutrients cows can take in is limited by the quality of hay or forage. The higher the quality, or digestibility, of the forage, the more nutrients are available. Lower-quality forages limit the amount of nutrition that a cow is able to take in before she has to stop and ruminate.

Dry matter intake (DMI) is a calculated estimate of how much the cow can take in of a particular quality hay or forage. It's based on years of observation and studies, and while there are a lot of things that can factor in, it's a reasonably close estimate and should work for our purposes. It's listed as a percentage of body weight in nutritional tables. (There are lots of nutritional tables on the Web, many from university-based agricultural extension services.)

So, let's say, as an example, we have a 1,000 lb. cow, just starting the first trimester of gestation. We have medium-quality forage, and our cow is not currently lactating. The amount of hay she will eat per day is 1,000 lbs. × 2%, so she will eat 20 lbs. of hay per day.

Next, we need to determine whether or not our hay will meet her needs. Consulting a nutritional table, we find that, at her current nutritional stage, she needs to eat 1.33 lbs. CP per day.

If our hay is 6% CP, she will be eating 1.2 lbs. CP per day, so slightly less than she needs. And, as she progresses in her pregnancy, her needs will increase.

At the last month of pregnancy, she will need to eat 1.88 lbs. of CP per day. So we need to figure out a supplement for her.

One of the easiest supplemental feeds for cows are cow "cubes," which are large pellets about the size of your thumb. They are generally high in protein, so it doesn't take much to make up the difference in diet.

If we have a bag of cubes that are 20% protein, and we need an additional .6 lbs. of protein daily, 3 lbs. of cubes will make up the difference (3 lbs. × 20% = .6 lbs.).

I'm math averse, and I break out into hives trying to figure nutrition...so I put a lot of energy into making sure I can get really good hay to start with. That way I don't have to do any more math than necessary!

Determining Energy

Our TDN from our hay analysis is 46%. Daily consumption of hay is 20 lbs.

20 lbs. × .46 TDN = 9.2 lbs. per day.

From nutritional charts we know that our 1,000-lb. cow needs 9.5 lbs. of TDN per day; so again, we are a little short with energy. Our 20% cubes will average about %70 TDN, and our 3 lbs. of cubes will more than make up the difference in energy (3 lbs. × 70% = 2.1).

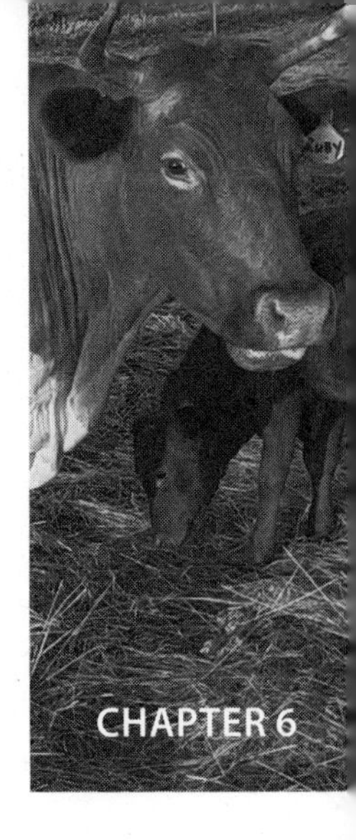

Reproduction in Cattle

Cattle are, of course, mammals—meaning they give birth to live young. These babies are *precocial*, which means they are born with their eyes open, are on their feet soon after birth, and traveling with their mothers very quickly. (By contrast, an *altricial* baby such as a baby rabbit, is born with eyes closed and spends its first few days in a nest built by its mother.)

Estrous in Cattle

Estrous is the term that refers to the entire cycle from ovulation through breeding to either a successful pregnancy or the next ovulation. Estrus refers to the actual period that the cow is willing to be bred and capable of conceiving. These two words have always been a little too closely spelled for comfort, so for purposes of this discussion, I'll use *estrous* to mean the entire cycle and *heat* to mean the period that the cow is ready to be bred.

The estrous cycle in cattle averages around 21 days. The range can span from 18 days to 24. Most individuals have a pretty precise cycle; if your cow has a 22-day cycle, she will generally cycle every 22 days.

Day one of the estrous cycle begins with ovulation. If the cow is bred and becomes pregnant, the cycle stops until the calf is born, and then begins again. If she does not become pregnant, the unfertilized egg is shed, and the process of egg development through ovulation begins again.

The heat period of the cycle is marked by the cow being willing to stand for the bull to mount her or, in his absence, allow other cows to mount her. Cattle in heat will also try to mount other cows. This period, as you might suspect, is called standing heat, and lasts about 18 hours.

The response to a cow in heat is so strong, that even pregnant cows will mount and ride other cows, although they will not stand to be mounted.

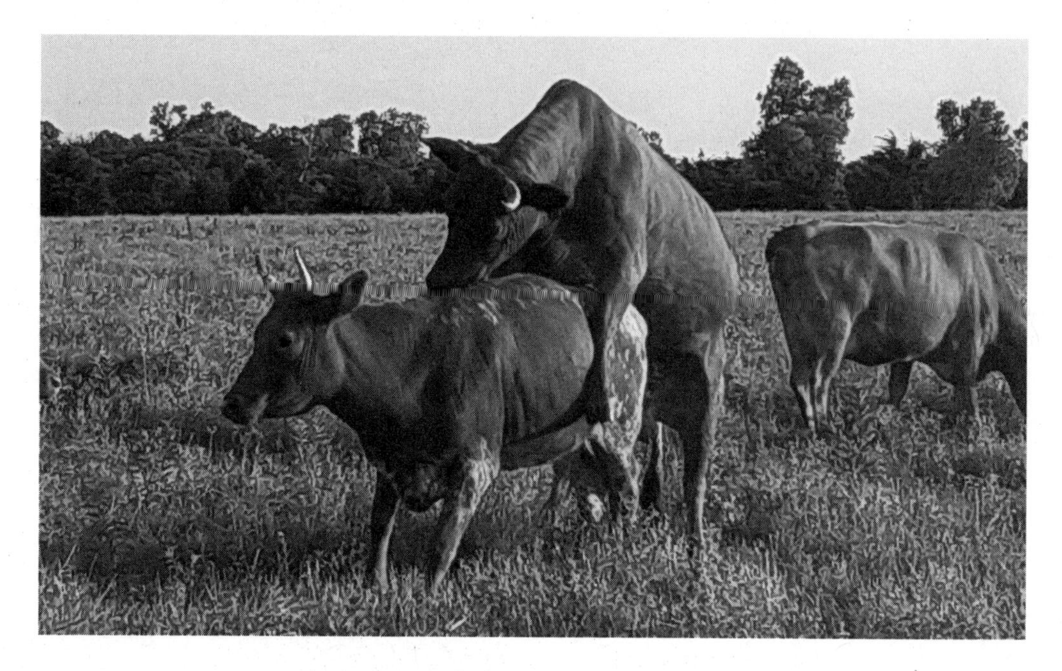

Cedar riding Effie.

Cattle are capable of breeding all year round. Other domestics have more of a season; horses are seasonally polyestrous and generally have a period during winter when they will not breed. Sheep and goats are the opposite; they tend to be more reproductively minded during the winter months. This helps those species give birth when the weather is generally more compatible and forage availability is approaching its peak.

This is something to keep in mind if you live in a climate where it would be a problem or a management concern to have calves in inclement weather.

If you are using a bull, it might be a good idea to remove him from the cow herd from March through June so that calves will not be born in December through February.

If you are using AI, just make sure to time the service right. You have a lot more control over the timing of calving using AI.

Freezing rain is harder on livestock than just about any other weather condition, and since February and March here in Kansas are often more than happy to serve that up, we try to avoid calving until after March.

Many commercial cow-calf operations want to calve as early as possible in the year to have the calves be bigger when marketed in the fall. Calves are hardy; once born and dry they tolerate cold weather well as long as they have adequate shelter from extreme wind chill

Calving Due Date Estimator

Bred Date	Due Date	Bred Date	Due Date
January 1	October 10	July 14	April 23
January 7	October 16	July 21	April 30
January 14	October 23	July 30	May 7
January 20	October 30	August 4	May 14
January 28	November 6	August 11	May 21
February 4	November 13	August 18	May 28
February 11	November 20	August 25	June 4
February 18	November 27	September 1	June 11
February 25	December 4	September 8	June 18
March 3	December 11	September 15	June 25
March 17	December 25	September 22	July 2
March 24	January 1	September 29	July 9
March 31	January 8	October 6	July 16
April 7th	January 15	October 13	July 23
April 14	January 22	October 20	July 30
April 21	January 29	October 27	August 6
April 28	February 5	November 3	August 13
May 5	February 12	November 10	August 20
May 12	February 19	November 17	August 24
May 19	February 26	November 24	September 3
May 26	March 5	December 1	September 10
June 2	March 12	November 24	September 3
June 9	March 19	December 1	September 10
June 16	March 26	December 8	September 17
June 23	April 2	December 15	September 24
June 30	April 9	December 22	October 1
July 7	April 16	December 29	October 8

and freezing rain. And cows are very good at finding places to stash their calf out of the weather. But for the small herd, it's not a huge amount of fun to calve in bad weather. So, time calving to work for your climate and your schedule.

Cattle have an average 283-day gestation length. There is some variance between breeds, but it's a close enough target for a due date.

If you have AI'ed your cow, you should be able to drill down pretty close to the due date. Don't become too alarmed if your cow calves either a few days before or after, unless she acts like she's having difficulty. Sometimes things take the time they take.

Pasture Breeding

If you don't happen to see your bull breeding your cows, don't worry. On our farm we rarely see anything happening but have had dozens of calves to prove the job 's been done.

In cattle, breeding happens pretty quickly, and the bull doesn't do a whole lot of courting before he gets down to business. I put a young bull in with a young heifer that was in standing heat one time, and he bred her six times in fifteen minutes. (I sent Eric a text play by play... He was thrilled.)

Bulls are described as contact breeders: once they're mounted and everything feels right, they will ejaculate and get down pretty quickly. And, as was the case with our young bull, in general bulls can breed multiple times in a short while.

Cattle are most easily observed in standing heat in the mornings and at twilight, and breeding most often occurs at those times, so it can be easy to miss.

Cows have a horned uterus: two separate uterine chambers joined by a short uterine body and a cervix. After the egg is

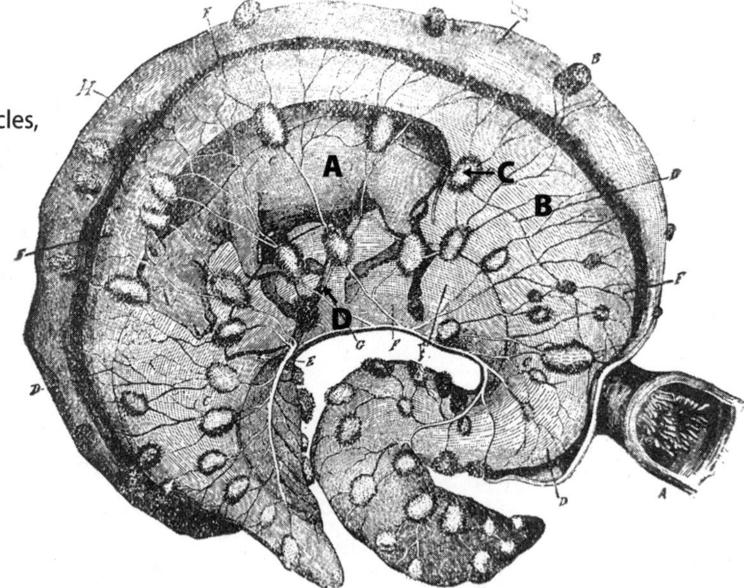

A Calf
B Amniotic fluid
C Placentome, caruncles, cotyledon
D Umbilical cord

Fetal membranes. The drawing is from The Veterinary Obstetrical Compendium *by Wales E. Van Ame, published in 1903.*

fertilized, the embryo will implant in one side or the other.

As the placenta is formed, it attaches to several points on the uterus. On the fetal side the attachments are called *cotyledons*; the maternal side, *caruncles*. These form points, rather like "buttons." Nutrients and waste are exchanged between the mother and fetus at these points. By contrast, in many other species, the placental attachment is described as *diffuse*, which means the entire placenta attaches to the uterine wall and exchanges nutrients and waste throughout most of the surface.

Twins are not unheard of in cattle, occurring only in about 1 out of every 200 pregnancies in beef cattle but higher at about 8 in 200 4% in dairy cattle. An interesting thing about cattle twins is that if the calves are a bull and a heifer, the heifer will usually be sterile. This calf is called a *freemartin.* Because the placental membranes are joined, hormones for each sex are exchanged and interfere with the development of reproductive organs in the heifer calf. The ovaries are very small, and the heifer will not show heat signs. The bull calf will not usually experience any fertility issues.

Puberty

Cattle reach puberty, on average, at 12–14 months. Of course, as with anything, there are exceptions either way.

Puberty is a function of nutrition, genetics, and management more than an exact date on the calendar. A complex system of hormonal controls and events are necessary for puberty to occur, and the conditions have to be right all the way round.

Percentage of mature weight seems to be a better indicator of puberty than age. Most heifers that have reached 65% of their mature weight will begin experiencing puberty. Heifers should be at 85% of their mature weight by the time they calve.

It's a common misconception that reducing the heifer's diet will reduce the calf size and thereby prevent calving difficulty. A heifer has to be extremely fat in order for calving ease to be affected. Reducing the diet just puts more nutritional strain on her, and makes it more difficult for her to rebreed after calving. In fact, failure to rebreed within 60 days of calving is the most common reason for young heifers to be culled from a commercial breeding herd. Make sure your heifers are physically mature enough to handle the strain of growing that calf, and give them a fair chance to earn her place in the herd.

Many heritage breeds, for example, mature physically a bit slower than commercial breeds. She may begin cycling at the average age but not yet be physically mature enough to carry a calf without overtaxing herself. Evaluate each herd

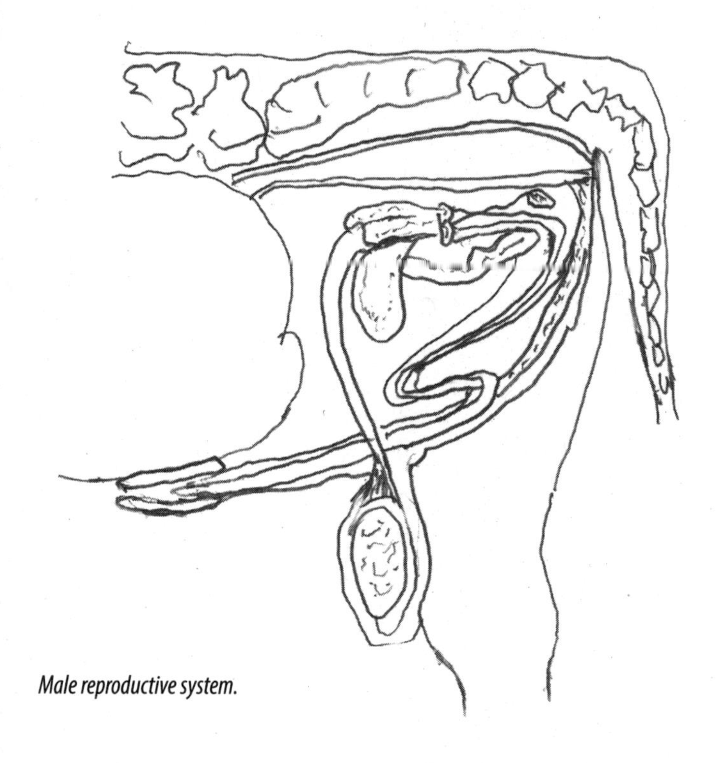

Male reproductive system.

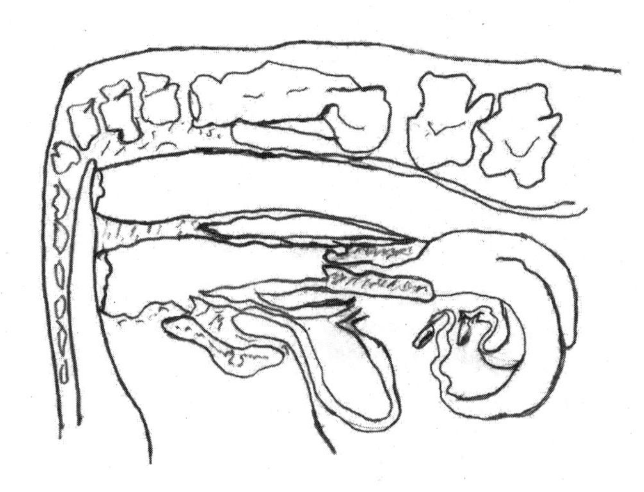

Female reproductive system.

and each cow as an individual and go accordingly.

Bulls can reach puberty at a younger age than females. The average is around 9–10 months, but of course exceptions can occur. It can also be confusing because bull calves will begin mounting their pasture buddies at a much earlier age and will often try to mount adult cows. As with females, puberty in bulls is related to age and body weight. In bulls the weight of the testicles is also a useful reference. Scrotal circumference is considered a highly accurate measure of scrotal weight. If a bull calf's scrotum measures 28–29 centimeters, you can generally bet he's starting to be fertile.

Although a young bull is capable of breeding, his fertility and reproductive capacity increases as he matures.

Artificial Insemination

According to legend, the first use of artificial insemination occurred centuries ago. An Arab chieftain wanted to breed a particular mare of his to the stallion of a rival. Using a rag soaked in mare urine to excite the stallion and cause him to ejaculate, he collected the sample, made off with it, and used it to inseminate the mare.

You have to wonder if this story is more fiction than fact, but somewhere, at some time, someone got the idea that it was possible to do something similar.

The invention of the microscope in 1677 enabled scientists of the day to see sperm cells, even though they weren't quite sure exactly what they were or how they functioned. It took another century before the first successful artificial insemination was performed, by Spallanzani, in 1784, in a dog. The dog delivered three pups. It was the end of the 1800s before there were reports of artificial insemination in rabbits, dogs, and horses, taking place primarily in Russia and other European countries.

In the 20th century, Russia led the way in developing AI procedures and technology, most importantly developing semen extenders (enabling several animals to be bred from one sample) and artificial vaginas, similar to ones used today. Previously, semen samples were collected from sponges placed in the vagina of mount animals.

In the 1940s, AI in the United States took off, and procedures were developed that became established worldwide. It was discovered that semen could be frozen in an egg solution and then thawed for later use. As cryopreservation methods were developed, long term preservation and storage of semen became routine.

AI brought major changes in the dairy industry. The collection and sale of sires selected for specific traits enabled breeders to make huge changes in the makeup of their dairy herds. AI became big business, and several large companies have grown up around it.

Even though AI is more common in larger operations, it can still have a place for the small herd.

Pros and Cons of AI

One of the major benefits of AI for the small herd is not having to maintain a bull. Bulls are great, but they have one job, and that's to breed cows. Otherwise, they just lounge around and eat.

Also, they can be dangerous. We've been blessed with very good-natured bulls over the years. But they can never be taken for granted. Even though they can be easygoing, if they perceive you as a threat or competition for their cows for whatever reason, they can become aggressive.

They can also decide to visit neighbor cows that might be in heat, which may or may not endear you to your neighbors.

If you have your bull turned out on pasture with your cows, you may not know due dates for your calves. And if you have cows with heifer calves, he'll breed the young heifers too, whether they are mature enough physically or not. If you don't want to have your bull living with the cows, you will need a separate pasture for him, with shelter, water, and a good fence, preferably reinforced with hot wire.

On the plus side for bulls, they will always know when the cows are in heat and ready to breed. A young bull will learn pretty quickly when a cow isn't in the mood and learn to behave accordingly.

A bull will breed the cow multiple times over the course of her heat period, and so, of course, the odds of a pregnancy go up.

The two down sides to AI are cost and heat detection.

AI equipment, nitrogen storage tanks and their maintenance, semen, training, and everything else that go along with the process cost money. They can be a long-term investment in your herd, but the up-front cost can be a turn off for a lot of people.

Accurate heat detection is probably the single biggest factor contributing to AI success. There are certain drug protocols that can be used to bring cows into heat at a specified time, but there are still a lot of variables.

Supplies needed for AI.

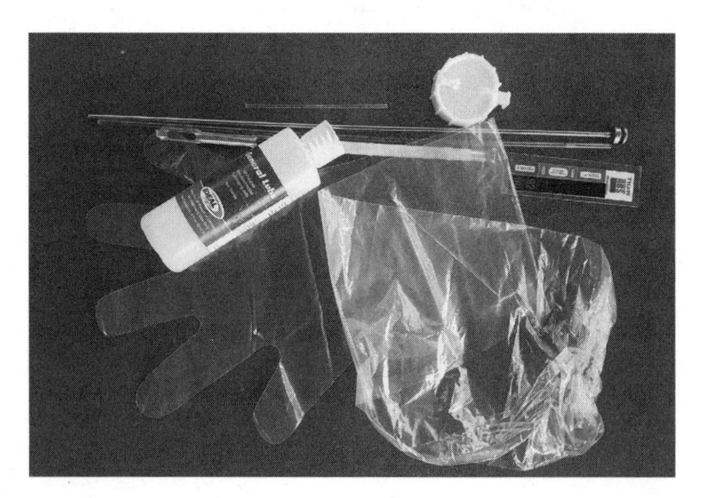

The up side for AI is access to bulls you might not have otherwise, and AI also reduces the potential spread of infectious reproductive diseases. Plus, no one has ever been charged in the pasture by a liquid nitrogen tank.

How AI Works

There are several companies in North America that specialize in collecting semen, holding it, and making it available to the public. They collect semen from elite commercial breeding stock producers, who have done a plethora of genetic testing on the animals, and can provide enough growth, carcass, and feed efficiency data to make your head swim. They publish sales catalogs with this information and a price list for the semen.

Fortunately, they also collect and store semen from less well-known breeds, which enables folks with heritage breeds to be able to take advantage of AI technology. Many companies will also custom collect and store semen for private individuals.

Some semen companies own the bulls they collect and store, but often the bulls are privately owned. If the company owns the bull, usually one payment can be made. If an individual owns the bull and the semen, payment is made separately to the owner for the semen and to the company for shipping.

Cattle semen is collected and stored in "straws." When purchasing semen, the price listed is per straw. Some companies will sell you a single straw of semen, but, with shipping charges, it makes more sense to buy multiple straws.

Semen is shipped in a plastic "goblet," which holds five straws, and two goblets are attached to an aluminum "cane." The semen is shipped in a small, well-padded container that is charged with liquid nitrogen vapor and will have a few days before it begins to thaw. You will need to either use the semen within a day or two of arrival or transfer it to your farm storage tank when it arrives.

Care and Feeding of a Liquid Nitrogen Tank

If you plan to use AI frequently, a liquid nitrogen tank is a good investment. They will last for years if properly maintainedand, if you do not have semen you need to maintain, they can be stored empty for quite some time.

An N_2 storage tank is a double-walled tank, with the nitrogen and semen stored in the inner tank and a vacuum between the inner and outer tanks that helps maintain insulation. The exterior of the tank is usually aluminum, which gives it durability.

If the vacuum between the inner and outer walls of the tank is lost, the tank will not stay insulated, so care must be taken in handling the tank. Don't bang it around, and store it off the ground to prevent scratches and scuffs, which can lead to microscopic holes in the exterior tank, or condensation, which can lead to corrosion.

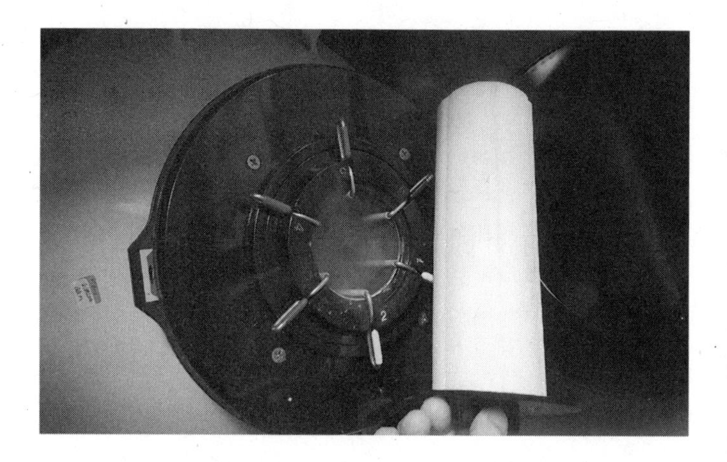

Liquid nitrogen tank.

Liquid nitrogen is a relatively safe element, as it will not explode easily, but at -320°F(-196°C) it can cause severe burns if it comes in contact with your skin.

The tank will have a narrow neck, which helps reduce evaporation of the liquid nitrogen. Liquid nitrogen vapors are nearly as cold as the liquid itself, so even if the tank is only half full, the contents will remain frozen. The length of time a tank will hold nitrogen depends on its size—a larger tank will hold more volume and be slower to evaporate than a smaller one. Nitrogen will evaporate faster if the tank is left open, so take care to make sure the Styrofoam cap is in place, and the lid is shut. Any tank must be checked regularly and have nitrogen added when it gets too low. If the tank runs out of nitrogen, the contents will thaw and be lost.

You can test the level of nitrogen with a specially made plastic stick (made not to shatter when frozen), available from most of the semen supply companies. Dip the stick into the liquid nitrogen tank, wait a few seconds and take it out. Frost will immediately collect on the stick wherever the liquid nitrogen touched it. Tanks will maintain a cold enough temperature to preserve the semen even with only a few centimeters of liquid nitrogen in them, but I make it a habit to never let our tank get below a third full. Having lived through a self-inflicted tank failure, checking regularly and keeping it on the fuller side just lets me sleep better at night. Most of the tanks will come with information about how many weeks you can expect them to stay full, but just because it says it should stay for 18 weeks doesn't mean it's a good idea to push it. Plan for regular refills.

Learning To AI

Artificial insemination is not complicated, but it can be complex. It is not something that you can learn well by just trial and error. Taking a class is critical for learning AI. Since 99% of the actual activity takes place inside the cow and out of sight, having someone coach you through what you are feeling is critical.

As AI has become much more common and widespread, several facilities now offer courses in the procedure. Many land grant universities also offer this training, sometimes as part of coursework, sometimes as an extra class that is open to the public. Also, your local extension agent can often be a resource to finding classes if that particular university does not offer a program.

The cost for this class is usually several hundred dollars, but don't be put off by the price tag. Good AI classes offer many cows to practice with and will give you several opportunities to practice. In the classes I've attended the only limit to how many times you can practice is how tired your arm gets.

The two AI classes I took over the years both offered an initial classroom session that went over the reproductive cycle of the cow, how to time AI, and various heat synchronization protocols. They also offered a look at a couple of cow reproductive tracts spread out on a table for you to get a look at exactly how everything appears and to practice passing an AI rod through the tract as it sits on the table. Make the most of this, because once you actually start with a live cow, everything is blind.

Most of the cows used in these classes are culls, just brought in for the purpose of this class. As the potential exists to damage the cow's tract by fishing around in unfamiliar territory with a stainless-steel rod, using good cows isn't a great idea. And often the reason some of these cows have been culled is they have had some reproductive issue, and their repro tracts are often...odd. If you can learn on these cows, when you go home to work on yours, it will often seem frighteningly easy and simple.

If learning AI isn't something you want to pursue, there are several other options. Your local large animal vet may provide the service. Most large animal practitioners have experience in AI, but unless cattle reproduction is a large part of their practice, they may not be practiced enough to feel comfortable trying. However, there is a good chance they will know someone who can do it.

Semen companies like ABS have people who are well trained and provide the service to their customers. Even if you do not purchase your semen from them, they may be able to AI for you. Their representatives are usually highly trained and experienced and up to date on the latest technologies.

A local college or junior college that has an ag program may also be a good resource to check. An instructor might have the skill or there might be someone he knows with the training and experience. Don't hesitate to ask around.

What to Expect

You'll learn all of this in your AI class, but this is an overview of what you can expect.

It involves feeling somewhat like you're threading a needle blind with your arm in a vise. Well, maybe not really, but it's not a super comfortable process. (And, honestly, it's probably more uncomfortable for you than for the cow.)

The first step is (with a palpation glove, of course) to reach into the cow's rectum. The bovine rectum is tough, to say the least. Other animals, such as horses, are much more prone to damage when palpating, but unless you are being unnecessarily insensitive and rough, the cattle rectum can tolerate your efforts.

The bovine rectum is also very, very muscular. As soon as your hand goes in, she's going to begin trying to push you out. This is entirely normal, and does not hurt her, but the pressure can be uncomfortable for your arm.

The cow's rectum is spacious enough that you will be able to feel her cervix, and pass the AI rod through the vagina into the cervix and deposit the straw of semen.

Rectal palpation is also how cows are checked for pregnancy.

Tips

Rectal palpation is probably not super comfortable for the cow, but I don't believe it's painful. Smaller cows that have never been AI'ed before may dance around a bit because it's a strange sensation. Some cows just plain don't like to be touched. Give them a few minutes to relax.

There's gonna be poop, y'all. It's gonna get on you. Wear sensible clothes and shoes.

You will need to "clean out" the rectum so you can feel the cervix, so just let that poop pass by, or if it's firm and dry, you may have to pull it out with your hand and go back in the cow. (Personally, I like to toss these poop balls at any watching hecklers.)

Use lots of lube. It makes moving your arm in and around more comfortable for you and the cow.

Pull that sleeve all the way up your arm, and it doesn't hurt to clip it to the shoulder of your shirt with a binder clip or a set of forceps. They also make a sleeve that has a tiny strip of rubber around the open end, which will help it stay up on your shoulder.

Heat Checking and Heat Synchronization

For success in AI, heat checking becomes important. Aside from good technique, the timing of AI is the most critical factor in success.

Heat Checking

- Plan to spend a little time observing your cows, morning and evening.
- Cows that are in heat will stand for other cows to mount.
- Cattle will go into a period of "standing heat," where they will stand for other cows to mount them, or they will try to ride other cows.

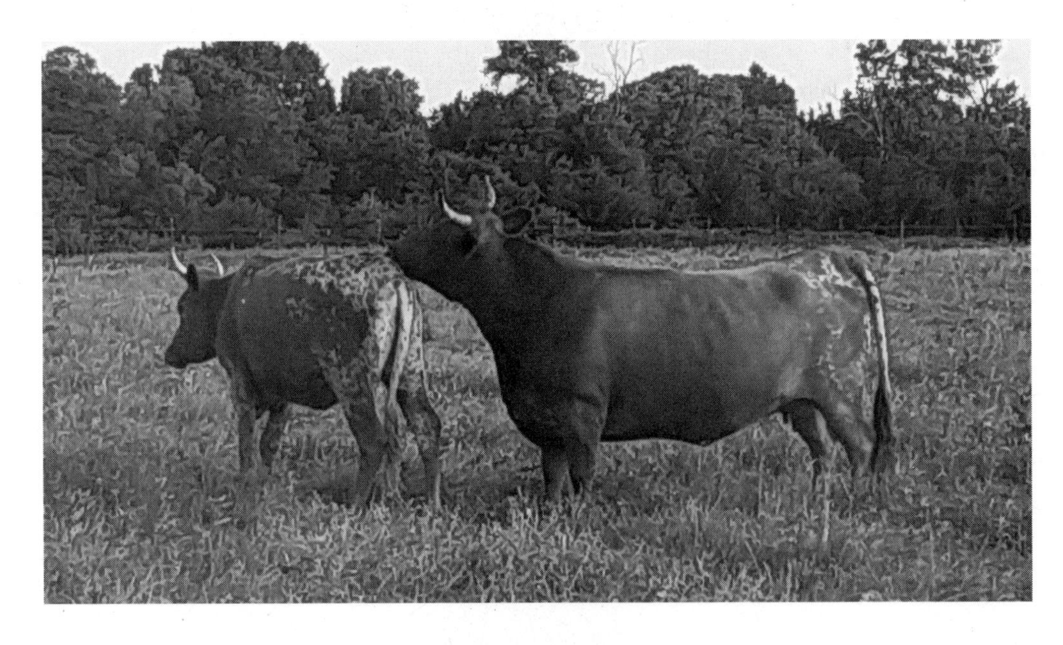

Cedar chinning Eleanor.

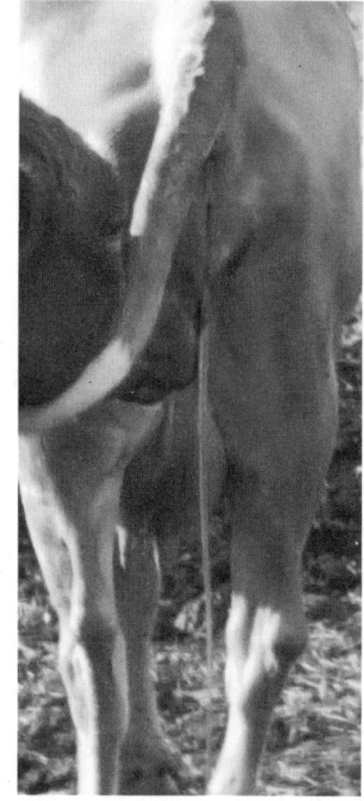

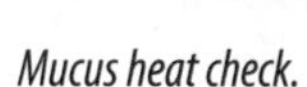
Mucus heat check.

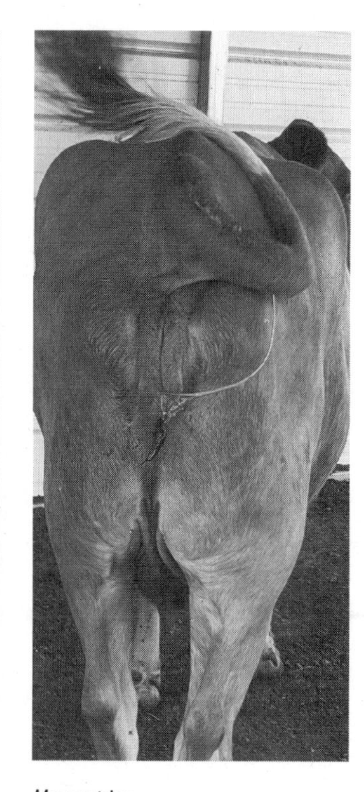
Mucus string.

- Riding happens fairly quickly. The key is to observe cows at least a couple of times a day.
- Most cows will show standing heat in the early morning and at twilight.
- Figuring the standing heat phase is 12–18 hours, cows spotted standing in the morning should be bred (AI'ed) in the evening, and cows observed standing in the evening should be bred the following morning.
- When we AI at home, Eric checks the cows first thing in the morning. Any cows observed in standing heat will be AI'ed that afternoon, after I get home from work. So far that strategy has worked well for us in our AI program.
- Decide when you want to calve, and then work backwards. Get an idea when you want to AI, and then give yourself a couple of cycles prior to that to make sure you know her cycle and can predict with a fair degree of accuracy when she'll next be in standing heat.
- While the average is 21 days, the range can be 18 to 23 days and still be completely within normal parameters. And be aware that heifers can have some variability within their own cycles, say 20 days one cycle, 21 or 19 the next, but generally not a huge variation along the lines of 18 days one time, 23 the next.
- That variability with heifers is one reason I like to spend a little time prior to when I want to AI to get a good idea of their timing. And, after a few cycles, even heifers get a consistent pattern.

Heat Synchronization

If you do not have the time or are not confident that you will catch cows in heat, there are a variety of drugs and drug protocols that can bring your cow into heat at a specified time.

I'm not going to go into them here. Your veterinarian or your ABS rep is the best resource for this information. New protocols and drugs are being developed

Heat Signs in Cows

Common heat signs	• Standing for other cows to mount. • Riding other cows • Clear, thick mucus discharge • Following other cows • "Begging"—turning around to look at a following cow—which indicates willingness to stand. • Vulva red and swollen • Chin resting on another cow (watch both to see which one is in heat-can be both)
Other signs that may or may not be seen	• Vocal, bellowing • Not interested in feed • Rubbed hair on tailhead from being mounted • Sniffing other cows and showing Flehmen response • Reduced milk production in dairy cows • Cows hanging out in groups
Post heat signs	• A streak of blood in the mucus—can occur 1–3 days post heat. Record that the cow was in heat prior, and watch for the next cycle.

Chart of heat signs.

all the time, and this is hard to keep up with if you don't work with them regularly. Many of the drugs require a veterinary prescription anyway; so start there.

Some of the protocols are complex and involve multiple injections, uterine implants, pulling the implants at a specified time, and so on, over the course of several days, and then inseminating at a specified time.

The more complex ones are geared for larger breeding stock operations, where it's possible (and part of the operations of the farm) to run cows through a chute multiple times to give the injections or whatever.

The simpler ones involve one or two injections.

Either way, you will have to be able to restrain your cow for the procedures, a couple of times at least.

Calving

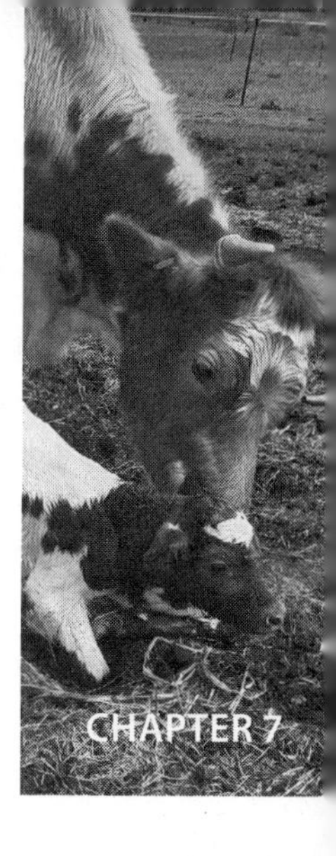

A WATCHED COW NEVER CALVES. At least that's the saying in our house. Cattle, and other animals, have a way of making you think that they are getting close to having their babies...only to give you another two weeks of sleepless nights worrying and checking and worrying again.

After several calving seasons, you'll start to get a feel for timing, and hopefully have fewer sleepless nights.

There are a few signs to watch for that can help you figure out when things are about to happen. One of the most visible signs of calving is that her udder will begin to fill up. And, just when you think it's full, it will get fuller. Depending on the breed and the individual, she may have what looks like a full, tight, ready-to-pop udder for some days before calving. The key to watch for is when the teats start to distend, fill up, and point forward. The pointing forward, also called "strutting," helps make it easier for the calf to find a teat and suck easily for the first time.

Her vulva will also begin to enlarge, and become spongy. This helps prepare the tissue for the stretching that's going to have to happen for the calf to make it into the world without tearing and ruining the cow's reproductive system.

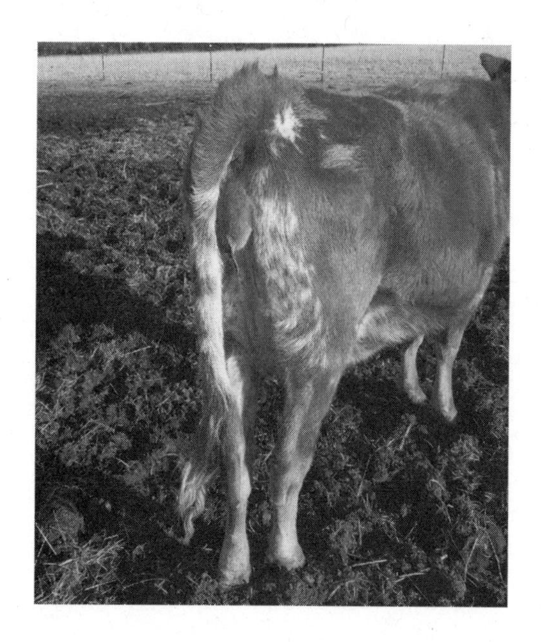

Relaxed tailhead. This cow calved the following morning.

The muscles around the tailhead will begin to relax, and the area between the head of the tail and the hipbones will become much more concave. This allows the ligaments to soften so that the calf can pass through the pelvis.

Her behavior may also change. She may become more secretive, start to isolate herself from the rest of the herd, and generally start to want to be alone. If you see a cow that's normally in the middle of the herd hanging out more by herself, it's worth keeping a close eye on her.

Cows tend to be pretty secretive about calving, but each cow is different. After a couple of calving seasons, you'll have a feel for what your individual cow's behavior patterns will be like.

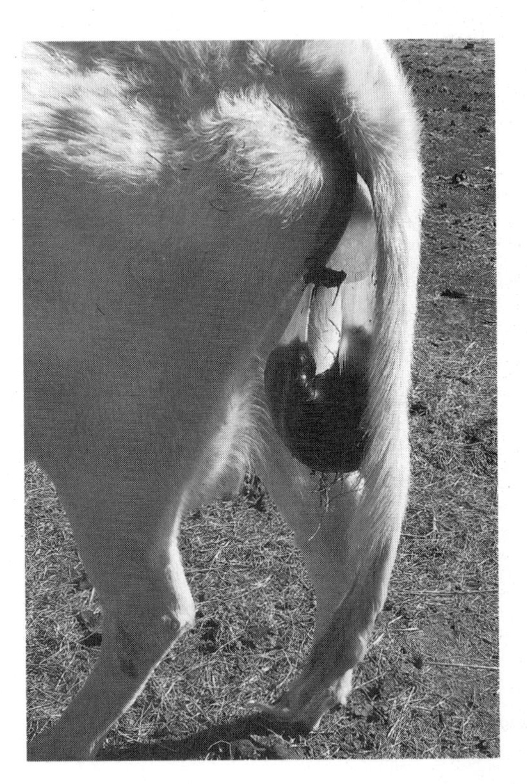

Allantoic sac.

Stages of Labor

The process of labor is divided into three separate stages, each with its own processes and events.

Stage One

This stage is mostly unobserved. During the 12–24 hours before calving, the calf moves around in the uterus, shifting from an upside down position to the front-feet first diving position that characterizes a normal delivery. The legs, which have been folded up while the calf is in utero, untuck and extend into the birth canal.

This is the time that her behavior may become more secretive. She also may be more restless, lying down and getting up frequently, just looking like she can't get comfortable. She also may urinate and defecate more frequently, as the calf makes room to move into the birth canal.

It's possible that you might see a contraction or two at this point, but they won't be very frequent or regular, and it's most likely you will not see anything, unless you are keeping a super close eye on your cow.

As the first stage progresses, you might see a "waterbag"protrude from her vagina. This is part of the allantoic sac and fluid surrounding the placenta and calf inside the cow's uterus. The fluid can be clear, or reddish, and will be watery. When this waterbag appears, she's moving out of stage one into stage two…: active labor.

Stage Two

This is the active stage of giving birth, the most visible, and the one most people picture when they think of calving.

This is where the cow gets down to business.

On average, this stage will take about an hour but can range from 15 minutes up to four hours.

This stage is characterized by visible, hard contractions. The cow will most likely be lying down, looking back at her rear end, and straining hard. Often her feet and legs will move as she pushes.

Previously, if you approached her while she's in stage one, she might jump up, give you a "Who, me?" look, and go back to grazing or head off to another location. But in this stage, things have progressed to the point where she most likely couldn't if she wanted to.

At this point, she's in a different mental zone, and it's possible to quietly approach her to watch the birth. Keep an eye on her reaction to you, though. If it seems like your presence is upsetting her, back off. Heifers, especially, don't have a real clue what's happening in their life right now, and they might be more reactive than an experienced cow. If she gets upset or stressed, the stress hormones might interfere with the process and cause delayed delivery or just make the whole process more difficult than it needs to be.

Normal Delivery

The calf should present front feet first, one slightly ahead of the other. The amniotic sac should be visible, or evidence that it has ruptured. The amniotic sac can contain up to 5 gallons of fluid, so it's pretty obvious. This is what's referred to as her

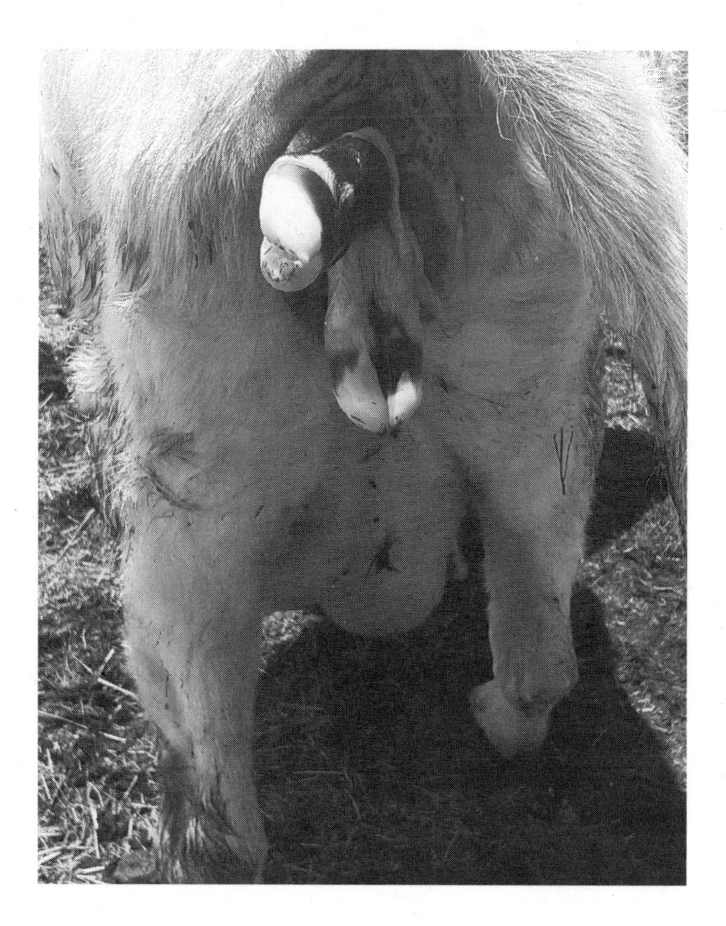

Feet-first normal delivery.

"water breaking." Often the amniotic sac breaks internally, and all you'll see is a flood of fluid being forcefully expelled from her vulva.

A normal delivery will progress steadily. Some cows take very little time to move the calf out into the world; others longer, but the key should be steady progress. Each time she strains with a strong contraction, the calf should move a little further out.

The front legs should be visible, with one a little further forward than the other. This keeps the calf's shoulders from trying to move through the pelvis at the same time, and allows one to pass through first.

The nose should be resting on the knees. Pushing the head through the vulva follows, and once the head is through, generally the shoulders follow quickly.

Once the head and shoulders are through, the cow may rest for a while with the hind legs still in the birth canal. This is perfectly normal and fine. If you are watching the birth, and the calf has

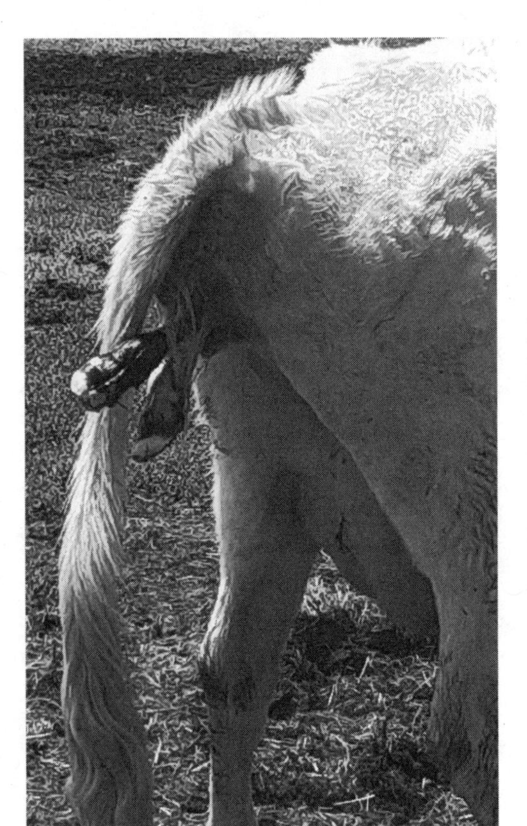

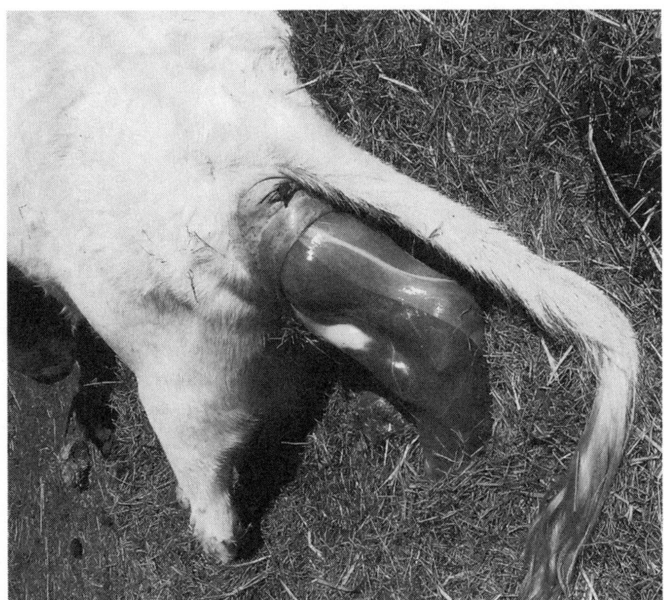

Left: *Feet further out.*

Above: *Head and front feet out.*

membranes covering his nose and mouth, it's fine to go ahead and remove those. The thin, fine, slimy membranes should not prevent the calf from being able to start breathing, but sometimes a thicker portion of the sac is still on the calf's face, and it always makes me feel better to go ahead and clear that off.

Check to see if the calf has begun breathing. (Let's say it's a bull calf, so *he* is the bull calf and she is the cow.) There is a reflex in place, while the calf is still attached to the placenta, that prevents him from taking a breath, so he doesn't drown during the birth process. Once his head and shoulders are out, he should begin breathing for himself. If he is not, you can tickle his nose with a piece of grass, pat him a little, and stimulate him to take that first breath. Then leave them alone for a bit—the calf will finish drawing the

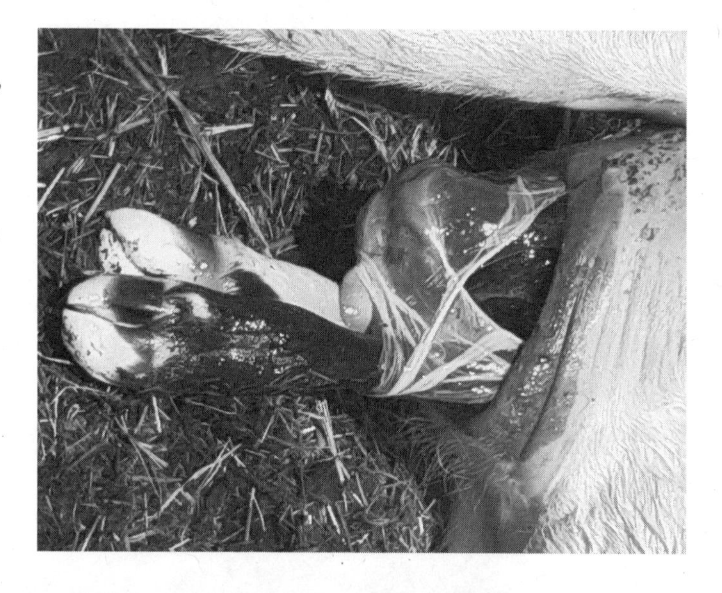

Feet and nose close up.

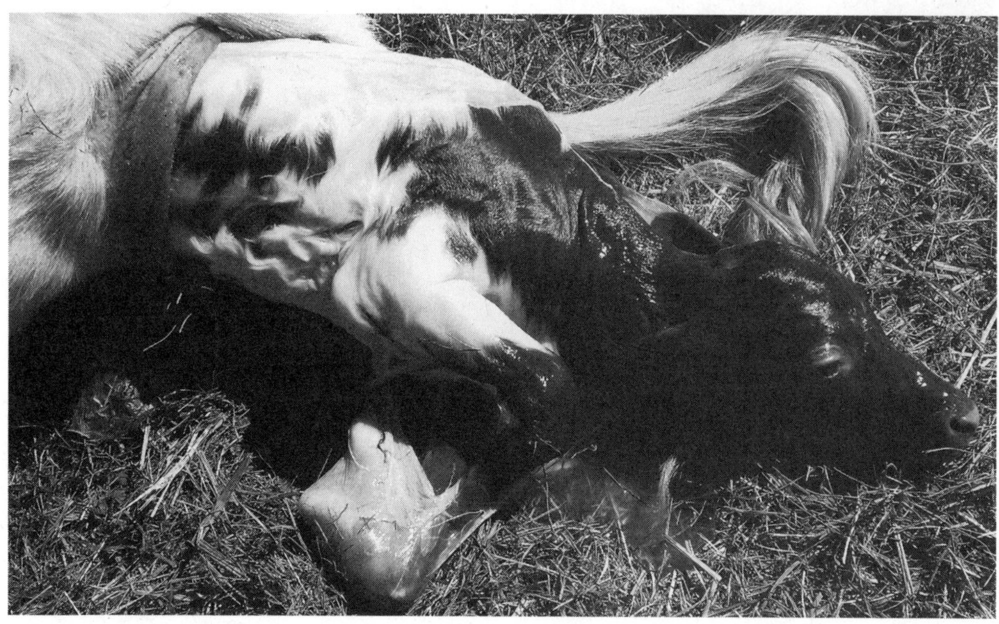

Shoulders and ribs out.

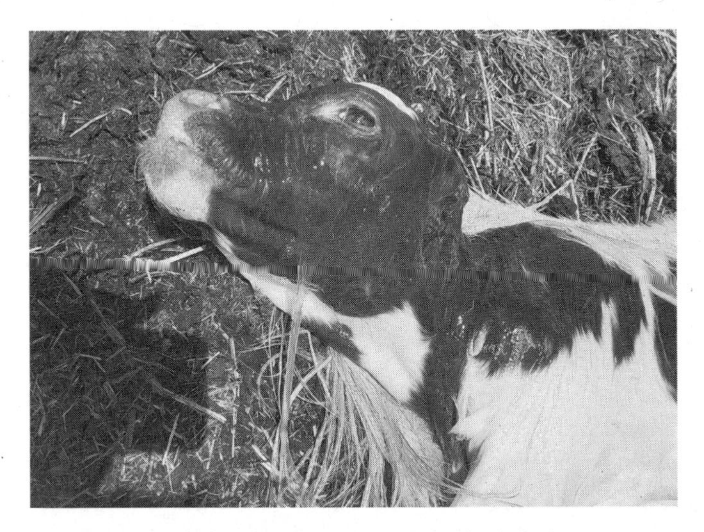

Live calf that has just started breathing, still coming to, after the birthing process.

majority of the placental blood supply into his own body.

After the major work of delivery is done and the cow has rested a few minutes, she should get up and begin to sniff and lick her baby. If the calf's torso or legs are still in the birth canal and she stands up, this will very unceremoniously dump the calf on the ground. It looks awful, but calves are pretty tough, and the stimulation of hitting the ground can help get the lungs moving and expel and fluids from the mouth or nose.

If the umbilical cord is still attached when this happens, it will stretch and break. Stretching and breaking on its own is best—this helps the vessels constrict

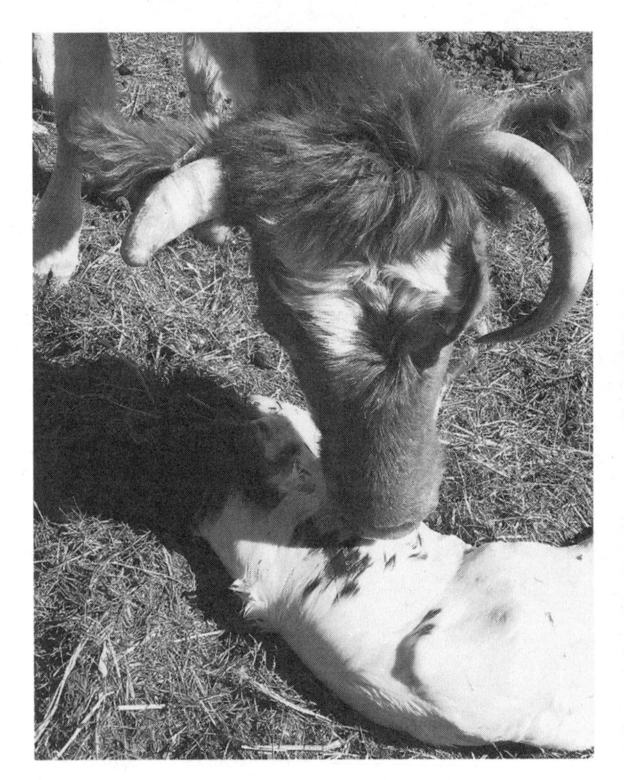

Cow licking calf.

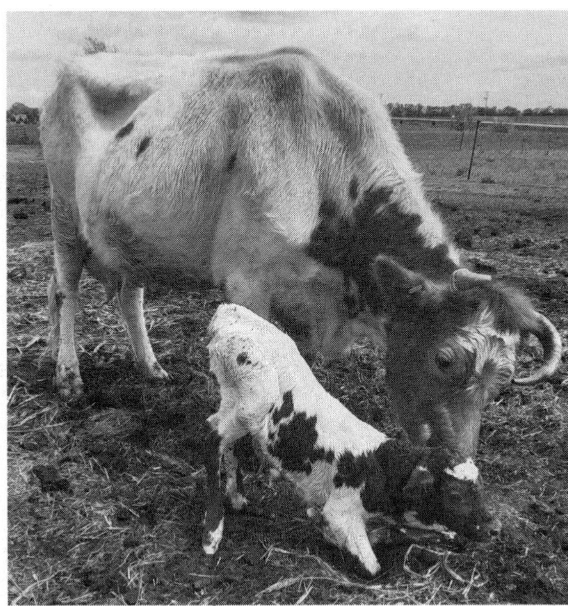

Calf getting up.

and shut down, whereas cutting it leaves open vessels that can lose more blood than is necessary.

Third Stage

The third stage of labor involves expelling the placenta and everything else that went along with the calf. She may strain a bit during this stage, but often the placenta slips out easily. The placenta should pass within a few hours of the calf's birth. If she doesn't pass it right away, try to find it when she does. The placenta is a rich food source for predators and there's no point in making things any easier for them. The cow will often eat her own placenta both to keep from drawing predators and also for the nutrition contained in it.

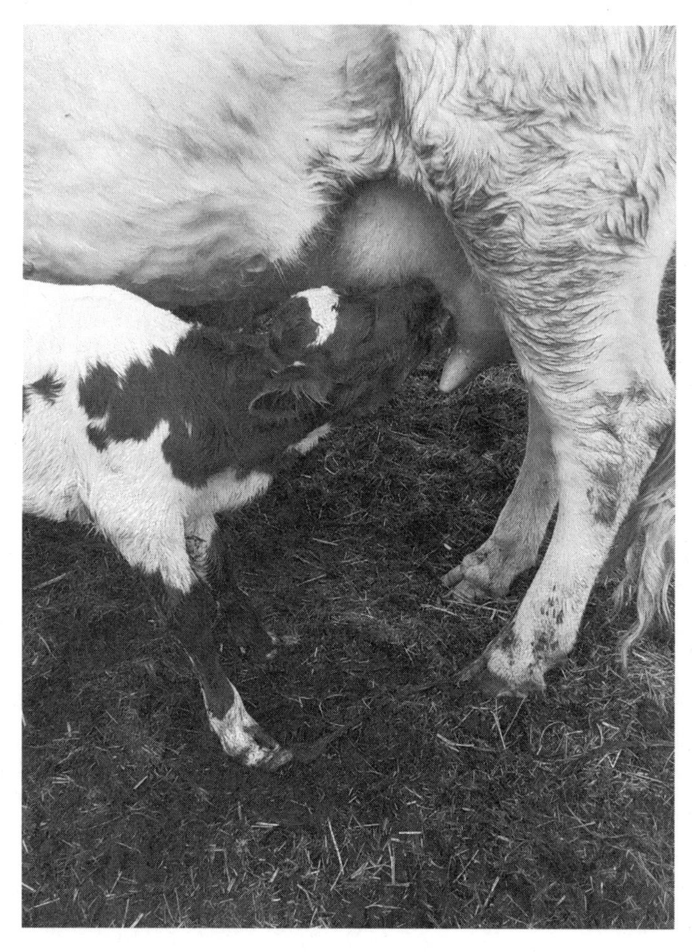

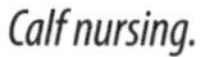

Calf nursing.

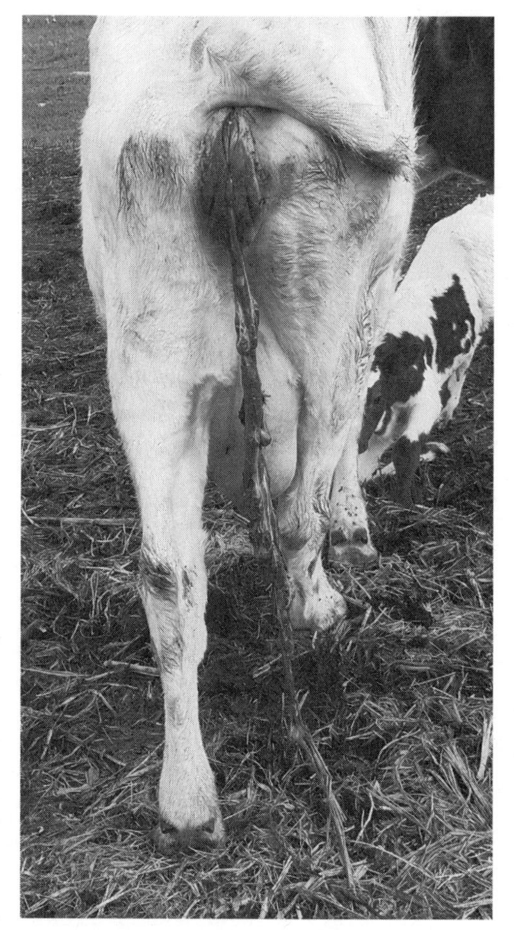

Placenta with cotyledons.

When Things Go Wrong...

If a cow has been in active, second-stage labor for an hour with no progress, it's time to intervene. The textbooks say an hour, but on our farm, with our easy-calving Pineywoods, if the cow hasn't made any progress in 20 minutes, I'm grabbing a sleeve and the OB lube.

Even if I called my vet and he dropped everything to run to my farm, he's still a half hour to 45 minutes away. The sooner I know if it's a simple problem that I can handle or a more serious one that I need expert assistance for, the better help I can be to the cow and calf.

An overly large calf is probably the most common calving issue. This is why it's critical to select bulls that are known for calving ease, in that their calves do not have a relatively high birth weight for the breed. With an overly large calf, the feet will appear to be in a normal position, the head might even be visible, but the cow can't make progress because the shoulders and the rest of the calf are too large for her pelvis.

Other signs of trouble are seeing front feet up to the knee with no sign of the head, or hind feet presented first.

Checking a Cow

Slip on your OB sleeve, and lube up. Squeeze your fingers together to make your hand as small as possible, and slip your hand into the cow's vagina. There's a lot going on in here at the moment, and she's actively trying to push things out, so be patient and work your hand in carefully. Feel around, and if what you feel seems abnormal, decide whether it's time to call the vet or if you are able to confidently handle the situation yourself.

If everything feels normal, with front legs and head in the diving position, maybe all she needs is a little more time. Heifers often take longer than cows. And if the calf feels overly large, she may just need a little help and traction to move things along. Sometimes a little gentle pull will do more good than using a lot of force, which can do more harm than good.

Simple Malpresentations

If both feet are coming out at the exact same time, instead of being one in front of the other, the calf can become "shoulder locked," meaning that the shoulders hang up on the pelvis. In this instance, just pull one foot further forward while pushing the other back slightly. This is usually enough to correct the problem.

If one foot is out and the other is not visible, reach in to see if you can feel the other leg. Most times the leg that is not visible just didn't get straightened out when the calf moved into birthing position. Push the calf back into the uterus and straighten the bent leg. (This is harder than it sounds since the cow

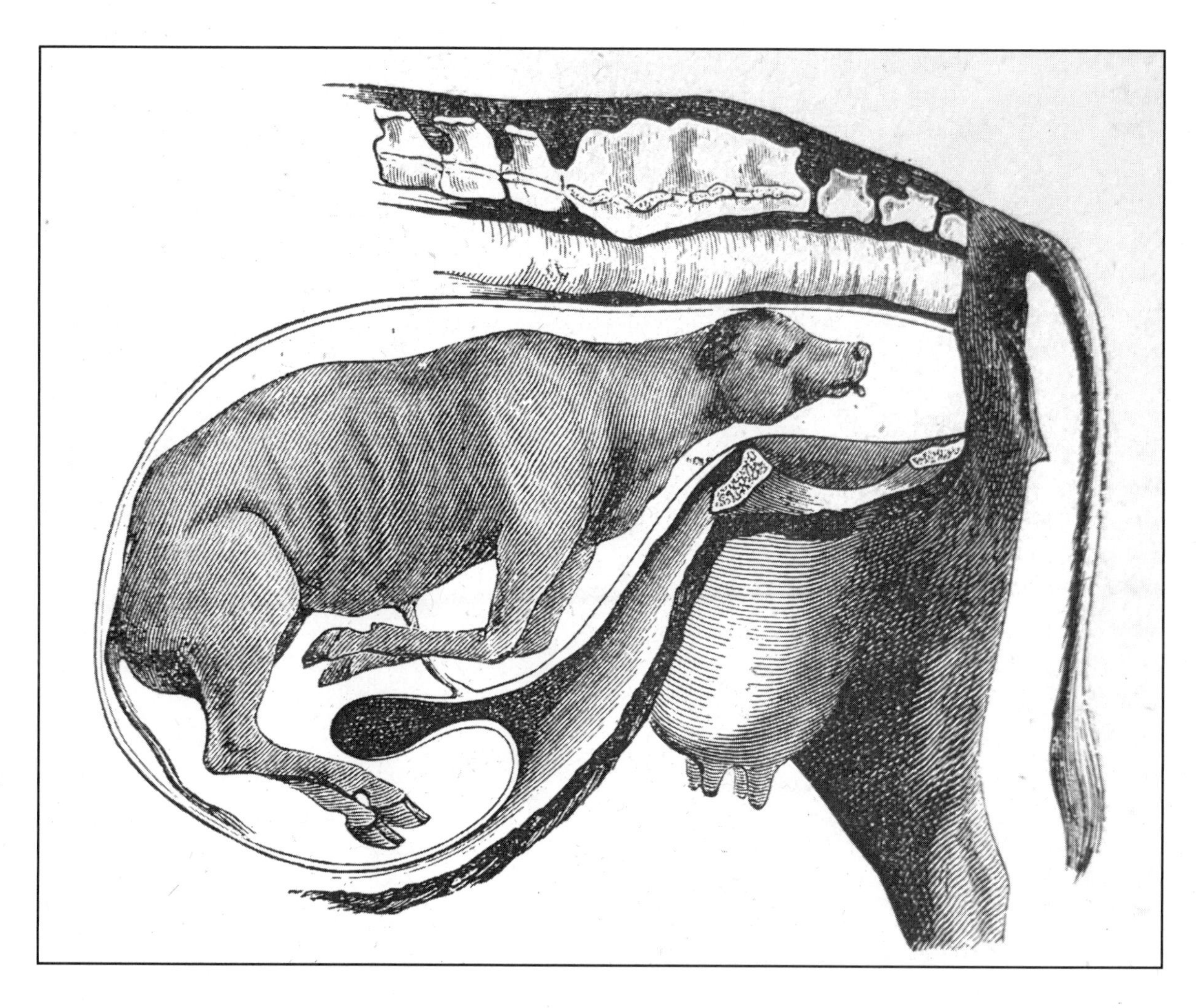

is still actively working to push that calf out!) Delivery should then proceed like normal.

Both-hind-feet-first presentation is generally not a problem, but often in a breech delivery the calf's legs do not extend into the birth canal, and she can't make progress with the calf. The solution is the same: the calf must be pushed back into the canal and the legs straightened out. Keep in mind, the calf is at a higher risk of suffocation during a breech birth, because the umbilical cord might become detached in all the maneuvering.

A calf with both legs and the head turned around is one of the most difficult to correct. It takes a great deal of effort

Forelegs not extended. The drawing is from The Veterinary Obstetrical Compendium *by Wales E. Van Ame, published in 1903.*

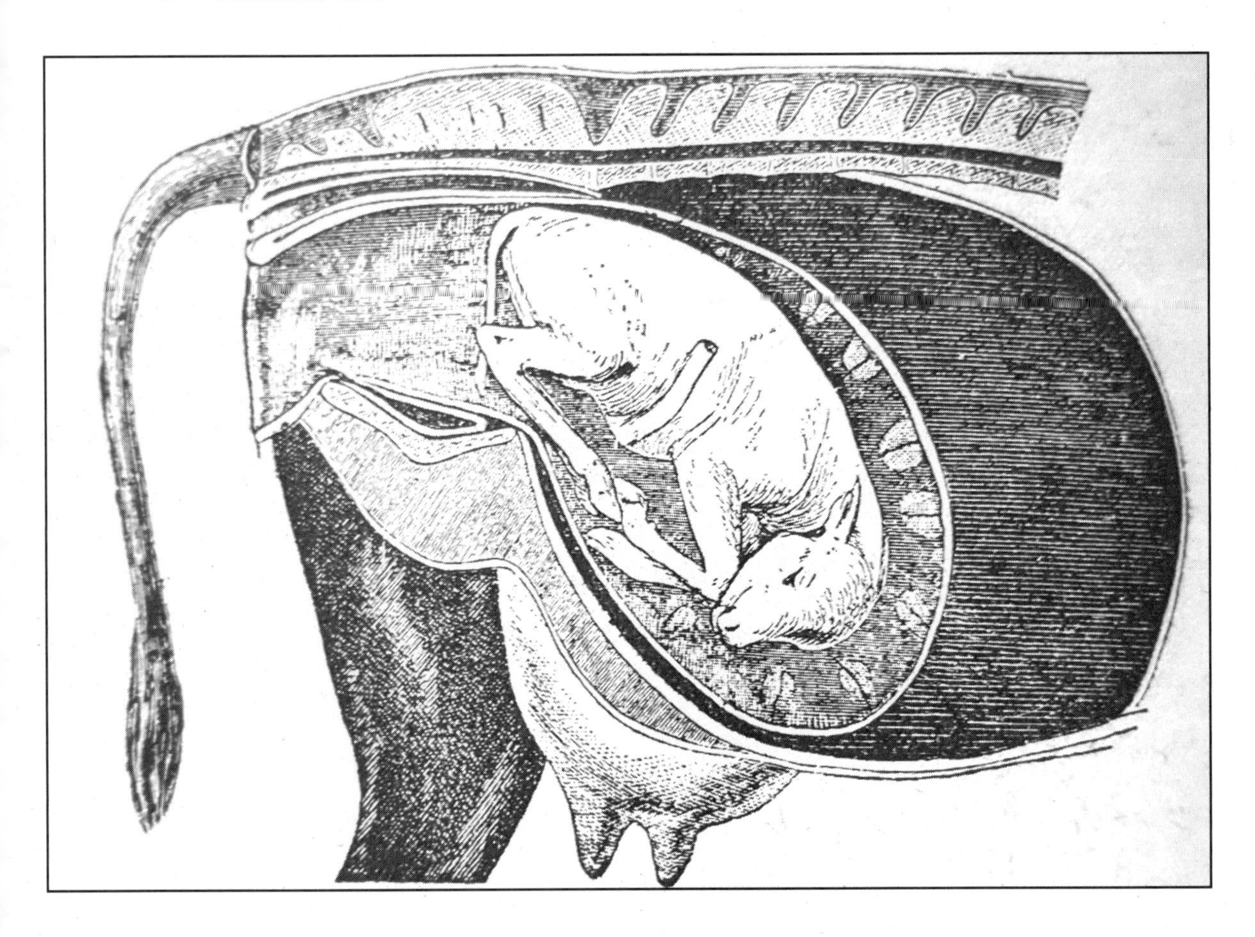

Breech. The drawing is from The Veterinary Obstetrical Compendium *by Wales E. Van Ame, published in 1903.*

to push the calf back in and turn the head. Often the cow's pelvis doesn't give you enough room to maneuver either. A calf's legs are pretty strong and can handle a strong pull, but in correcting this malpresentation the easiest thing to get a grip on is the jaw, and that can be easily dislocated and damaged or broken. You must grab the entire muzzle of the calf and there isn't a lot of room to work. This is a delivery that often does not have a successful outcome without timely intervention, and sometimes even then there is not a happy result. The cow gets exhausted; the stress of the delivery takes a toll on the calf; and often just the length of time the cow is in labor results in death.

In the years we've had our Pineywoods, we've had only one instance of having a problem delivery. Guess which kind of delivery it was. Yep. The hardest one. A quick check of the cow showed legs and no head, so we moved

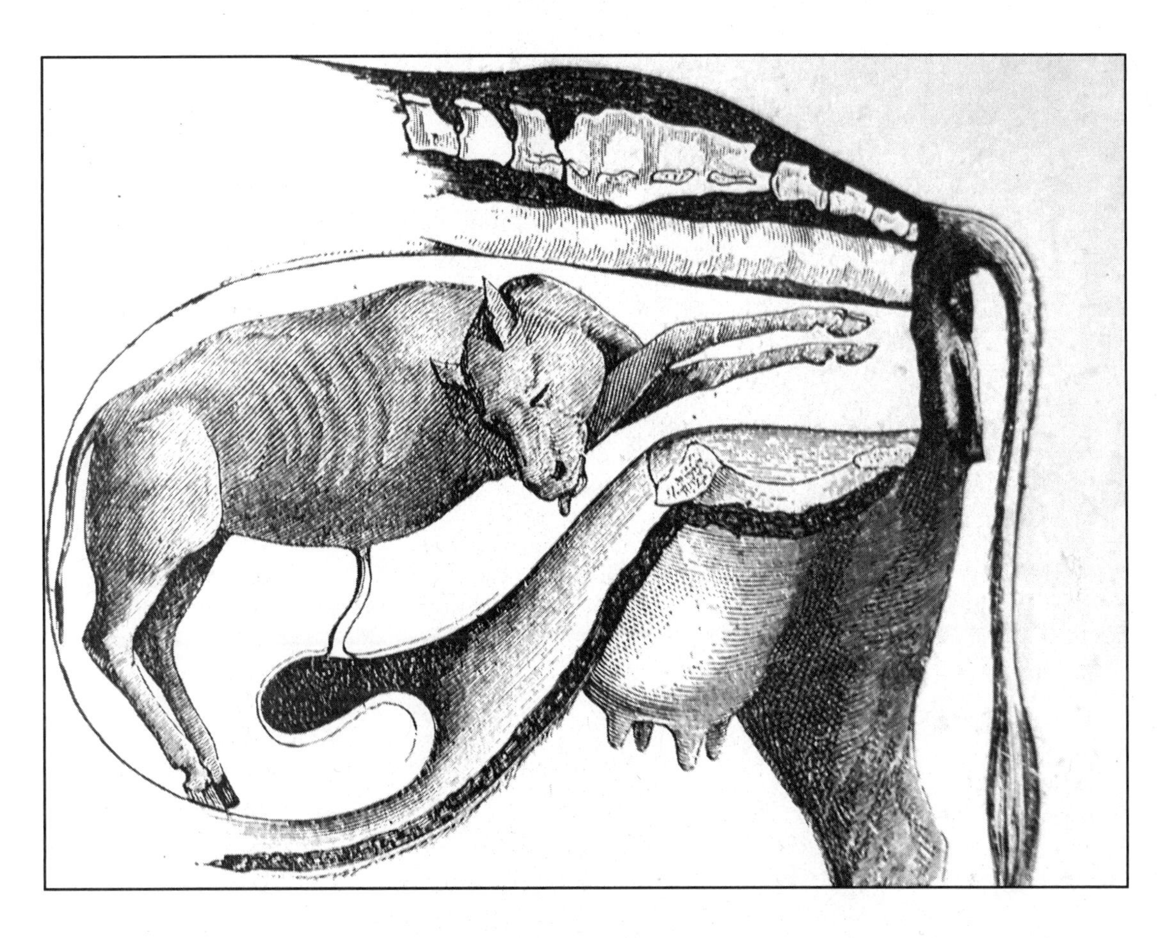

Head turned back. The drawing is from The Veterinary Obstetrical Compendium *by Wales E. Van Ame, published in 1903.*

the cow into the chute right away. I can't even describe how challenging it was to get both arms in that cow and push and move things around until I got that calf's head back around. My arms aren't huge, which helped me have a little room to work, but they're short, and just as I would get her pushed back far enough, I'd run out of grip on the cow. We worked for probably 45 minutes to an hour, and just as I was about to give up, the head slipped around and we were able to get the calf out. And then call off our vet, who I had figured was just going to help extract a dead calf, in pieces.

The calf was alive but exhausted. Both the calf and I were covered in the yellowish fluid that occurs during a stressful delivery.

I figured mom would be too stressed and exhausted to even care about the calf, but once she was let out of the chute she went to work cleaning up her calf and taking care of him. I tell you that story not to scare you, or brag on my calving abilities (because I do believe there was a little divine intervention there) but to illustrate that if there is any question or concern about a calving: *call the vet*. Nobody likes vet bills, but a dead calf and/or cow is worse. The story is also a reminder that a chute or some means of restraining a cow is absolutely necessary to have on hand.

Restraining a cow becomes necessary in the case of the most difficult malpresentations. A headgate or chute or, in the case of a calmer cow, a halter and rope, or a barn corner in which you can push her against a wall will be a necessity.

Eponychium shortly after birth.

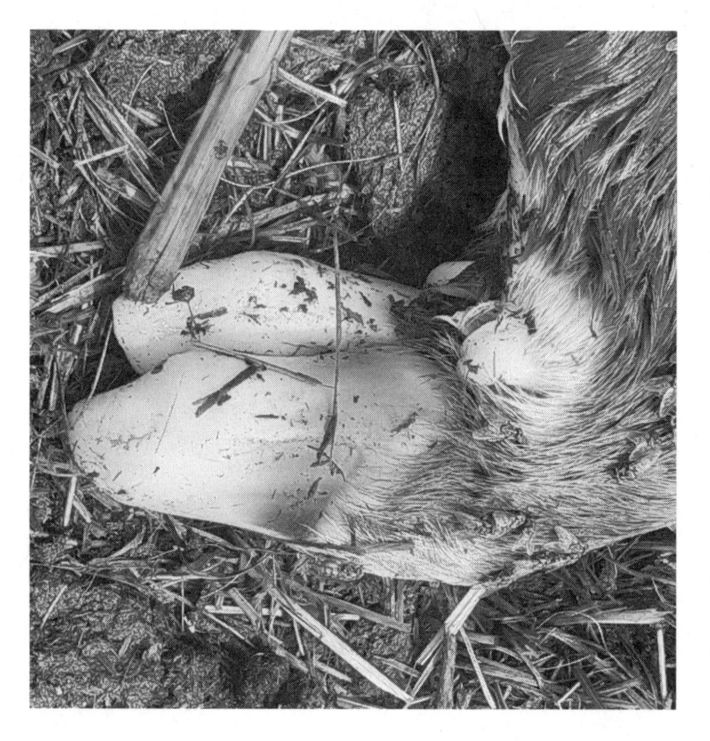

After a Difficult Delivery

The cow and calf are going to be exhausted. Once she's free of the chute or headgate, put the calf under her nose, and let them both rest.

It is entirely possible that she won't want anything to do with her calf, but give her a little time and, while she's resting, make a plan for bottle raising the calf. If your luck is like mine, if you make a plan for something, you won't need it.

It is also possible that, after a difficult delivery, it may be more difficult for the cow to conceive and carry another calf, depending on what sort of damage was done to her reproductive tract.

In my case, I figured that after all the time I spent crawling around in her uterus, with what felt like both arms and both feet at times, she was never going to calve again.That was disappointing, as she was one of my favorite cows. She took a year off and then, just as I was thinking about who I needed to cull, she presented me with a beautiful heifer calf. As one of my favorite vets likes to say, "Tincture of time does wonders."

Have you ever wondered how hooves don't damage the cow's reproductive tract on the way out? Mother Nature has fixed that with the eponychium, or the "slipper" that encapsulates the hoof and dries up and wears off shortly after birth. All hooved mammals seem to have them in one form or another.

Post-Calving Problems

Retained Placenta

One of the most common post-calving problems is a retained placenta, which is what happens when part or all of the placenta does not pass within about 12 hours after calving.

In the not-too-distant past, the recommendation was to help the cow clean out, either by attaching weights to the hanging placenta to help provide traction or to physically remove the tissues.

Recent studies have shown a better likelihood of the cow recovering if things are just left alone. The cow's uterus is designed to clean itself out, and while it's certainly not pleasant to see, eventually the tissue will liquify and pass on out, and she'll rebreed, although it might take an extra heat cycle.

It's not uncommon for a cow to have a discharge for a few days after calving, or for her to not have a discharge immediately after calving but then have a slight discharge 10 days to 2 weeks post birth. Both of these are just part of the healing process the uterus goes through. But if the discharge is excessive or foul smelling, or if she acts "off" and has a temperature, have the vet check her out.

Mastitis

Another possible problem is the cow having mastitis, which is an inflammation and infection of the udder, making her milk unsuitable for human consumption due to the high bacteria counts. The milk is still safe for the calf, though. It is more common in high-producing dairy breeds, and can affect one or all four quarters. Her udder will look and feel inflamed to the touch and be tender. Her milk will also not flow freely. A mild case might be cured by keeping her milked out well, but most likely she will need an antibiotic injection, and an antibiotic infusion that goes directly into the udder via the teat canal. As always, it's best to consult with your vet for advice. If a case of mastitis is not cleared up, she can continue to have problems, and her udder can be damaged.

Calf not Nursing

There can be several reasons a calf might not be able to nurse right after birth.

If the cow's udder is extremely distended, or she has extremely large teats when the udder is filled up, the calf might not be able to get his mouth around the teat and be able to provide the suction needed to get milk flowing.

In the hours preceding birth, when the udder fills up with milk, a waxy plug of sorts will form at the end of the teat canal. This keeps milk from streaming out onto the ground, but it can sometimes be firm enough that it doesn't dislodge when the calf first starts to nurse.

In either of these cases, you will need to milk the cow out to relieve some of the pressure so the calf can succeed when he tries to suckle.

Save this colostrum! This stuff is liquid gold. Freeze it in a freezer-proof jar or bag. Label it with the cow's name and date. Should you have a problem with a calf in the future, this colostrum can save another calf's life. It will have antibodies from your farm and be many times better than a general colostrum replacement you can purchase.

A calf that is not getting anything from the udder will be restless, trying each teat to see if he can get some satisfaction. He will head butt the udder, trying to get things flowing. Ultimately, he will get discouraged and quit trying, and if you don't intervene he will go downhill rapidly. And while a calf that is getting milk will also do those things, there is a restlessness, almost a desperation, in the behavior of the calf that is not getting a full tummy.

When a calf is latched on to a teat and milk is flowing, he will remain on the same teat for a few minutes, and sometimes you can even hear slurping noises. Most of the time you will also see an excited little tail wag.

Of course, just to confuse things, it can take a calf what seems to be forever to get latched on to a teat even if everything is fine. They bump around and attempt to suckle on everything but the udder. This is perfectly normal. As long as mom is not actively trying to kick him away, give him a few minutes and see if he figures it out.

Colostrum is much thicker than regular milk, so don't be alarmed if it doesn't seem that there is much volume. The higher energy and fat content of the colostrum will get him through the first few hours.

If your cow is tame, check to see if milk is flowing freely. If she's not tame, and you are concerned, put her in the chute or restrain her, and check the udder.

If a calf has nursed, often one quarter will be noticeably less inflated than the others, and often there is evidence that he's nursed by hair on her udder being matted from the calf's saliva.

You can also check the calf's tummy to see if it's full. Grab him and feel underneath, between the ribcage and the back legs, in the flank area. If he's had a good meal, this area will feel full and firm. If not, it will feel more hollow. It can be a hard distinction to make unless you've had a chance to feel the difference a few times, but if his tummy feels less than full, combined with some of the other evidence he hasn't nursed, it may be time to intervene.

In the case of a difficult delivery, the cow may be exhausted, sore, and not interested in her calf. I'm always a big fan of giving them some time and space in that instance, but if the calf hasn't nursed within 2–4 hours, I will do something to get some colostrum in his tummy right away.

If your cow is still lying down, it's possible to milk some colostrum out before she gets up.

When giving the colostrum to the calf, I've had decent luck using a 12-cc syringe, letting the calf suckle on my thumb or finger, and then letting the colostrum run down my finger into his mouth. You don't want to shove the colostrum down his throat—he can choke or aspirate and that can cause even bigger problems. Also, you want to make sure he knows that suckling is what makes the magic happen. Give him as much of this as you have and as he wants to take.

Colostrum is rich enough to get the calf through the first 12–24 hours, but if he is still not nursing you will need to decide what your plan should be.

When to Rebreed

The cow is pretty much designed to have a calf a year. A nine-month gestation, combined with a 60–90 day period for her uterus to heal and get back in shape gives you an annual calf.

About 45 days after calving, she will have her first heat cycle. The general wisdom is not to try to breed on this cycle, as the conception rate is much lower. The second post-calving heat cycle usually has a higher conception rate and has given her that extra time to heal.

If your goal is to get a calf a year, and to have that calf come at a certain time, you'll have to stick pretty close to that 60–90 day window. If you're more flexible on time, giving her another couple of months won't hurt; just be aware that she'll be in peak lactation three months after calving, and depending on her level of milk production, the extra strain of maintaining that level of production might have an effect on breeding success.

Calving Season

In a commercial herd, the goal is to wean as heavy a calf as possible in the fall; therefore producers try to get their calves on the ground in the late winter months, usually February.

If you don't live in a southern climate, February can come with some of the nastiest weather of the year. Once a calf is born and dried off, it can handle colder temperatures, but a cold rain, sleet, and high winds can be deadly. Winter calving will require some sort of shelter for the cow and calf, be it a barn, run-in shed, or a dense stand of trees.

The one plus of a winter calf, other than the heavier fall weight, is no insects!

Calving in late spring and early summer can take advantage of peak forage, and the weather should be milder. The tradeoff is insects, and as a newborn calf doesn't quite have the ability to regulate his body temperature, heat can be a problem.

Fall calving has gained popularity in some areas over the years. The cow should be in good body condition coming off summer pastures, and themarket for calves in the spring may bring higher prices, since the supply will be lower. The disadvantage will be that the cow must be provided with good-quality nutrition through the winter, either in the form of high-quality hay or supplementation with cattle cubes or grain. If she does not have good winter nutrition her condition may drop and lactation and rebreeding may be a problem.

There's no one right time of year to calve, just factors to take into account with every time of year. We've settled on April or May here for the bulk of our calving, and a second smaller crop in October. This lets us split the difference between avoiding the inevitable late spring ice storm, making the most of summer grass, and not having to spend too much money on extra feed in the winter. I think we've had a calf in every month of the year. Keeping a close eye on a cow due to calve, and having a plan in case the weather is unfavorable, have gone a long way in contributing to our success.

Care of the Newborn Calf

Colostrum

Besides protection from the elements, a healthy meal of colostrum is the most important first thing for the calf.

Colostrum is the first milk that the cow produces. It is thick, creamy colored, and high in energy and fat, and it contains essential antibody protection that the new calf needs. If the calf misses this meal, he will be at risk for every infectious challenge the environment can present. The energy and the fat in the colostrum will also help him get off to a vigorous start. Because it is so rich, the calf may nurse only a few times in the first hours of life, but the initial meal of colostrum is critical.

The cow will produce colostrum for two or three days post calving, but the calf can absorb the antibodies well for only the first eight hours. After that the ability to absorb drops off dramatically, and after 24 hours is nearly nonexistent.

Calves that do not get adequate colostrum are at a much higher risk for death in the first two to three weeks of life. Without the passive transfer of immunity provided by colostrum, they have no defenses against pathogens in the environment.

The best sight in the world immediately after calving is seeing the calf up and seeking the udder. Sometimes it looks like they are never going to quite get the hang of it, but once they get latched on and nurse well, they're off to a great start.

It's usually pretty easy to tell if they are latched on and milk is flowing. If the calf seems to be nursing but then stopping, head butting the udder, switching from side to side, and never latching on for more than a few seconds, it might be a good idea to check the cow's udder. Sometimes if the teat canal is plugged the calf can't nurse aggressively enough to get it clear and flowing. Milk a couple of squirts out of each quarter and stand back and let him try again.

A calf that has nursed adequately will have a plump tummy, not feel or appear hollow in the flank area, and not be actively seeking to nurse from anything and everything it comes in contact with. Another good sign that a calf has nursed is seeing meconium. Meconium is the first stool, and it's usually a black, tarry-looking substance. Seeing it is a good indicator that the calf has nursed and the digestive system is working.

Navel Stump Care

Treating the navel stump with a solution of iodine or chlorhexidine is also a good step. When still wet, the navel cord is basically a wick up into the body cavity of the calf. Dipping the navel stump keeps that area clean and minimizes the potential for infection.

If your cow calved in a clean, grassy pasture this is not quite as critical, but if she calved in a dirt lot, or an otherwise less clean area, it's best to try to get it done.

Chilled Calf

Once they are dried off, calves are surprisingly cold hardy. But if they continue to be wet, or born during a cold rain, they may become chilled. Get them out of the wet weather into a barn or shelter. Dry them off with towels (it's a good idea to keep a stash of old towels handy for just this purpose) or handfuls of dry hay or straw. Let the cow lick them to help dry them and stimulate circulation.

If they are extremely cold, they may become lethargic. In this case it may be necessary to move them into a heated room, or submerge them in a tub of warm, not hot, water. If you do decide to go the warm-water route, don't leave the calf unattended. If it is very lethargic, it won't take much for it to slip underwater and drown.

Calving Kit

These are all basic items in our calving kit. A small toolbox works great for storing the items, keeping them clean, and making them harder to misplace.

- Iodine or Nolvasan
  For disinfecting navel stumps and cleaning equipment
- Dip jar
  For treating navel stumps
- Thermometer
  for taking temperatures
- Bulb syringe
  For cleaning mucus and fluids out of the nose
- OB gloves (shoulder length)
  For assisting deliveries

- Lube
  For palpation, or delivery assistance
- Halter and rope
  For restraining cow if necessary
- Flashlight
  Because the difficult ones rarely happen in broad daylight
- Towels
  For drying the calf, or yourself if necessary
- OB chains
  Invaluable for helping assist deliveries

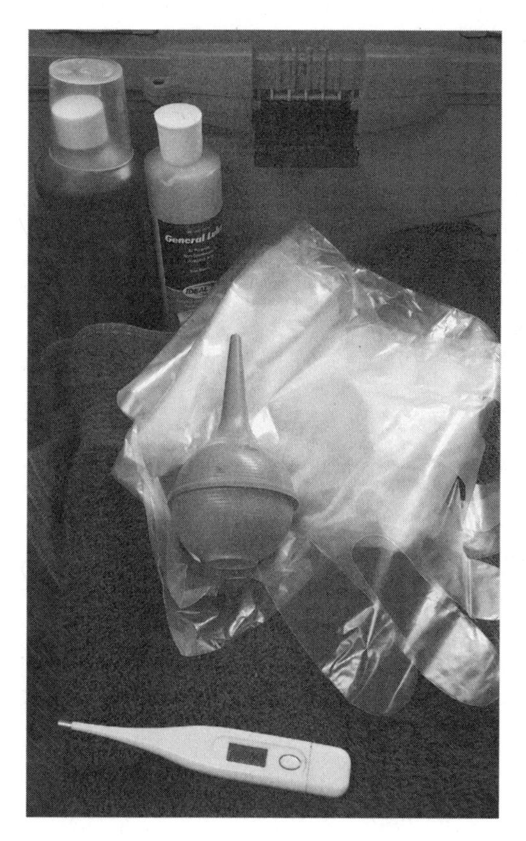

Calving kit.

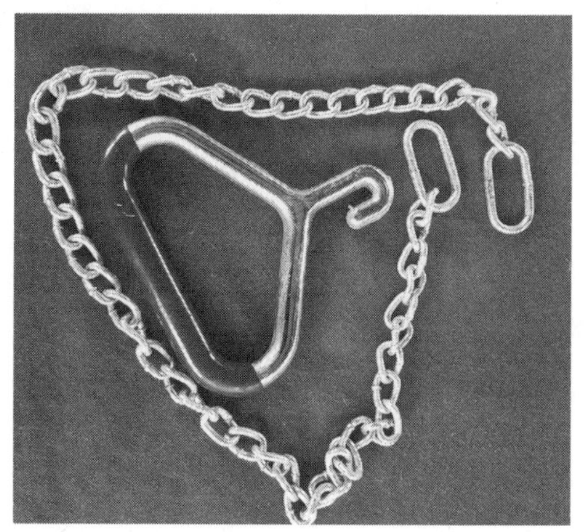

OB chains.

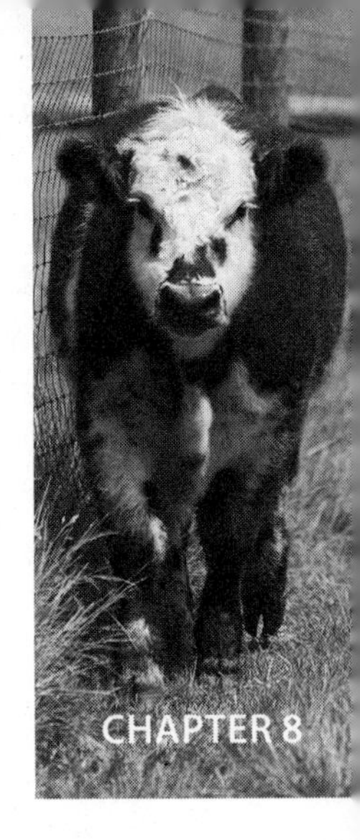

Raising Calves

If Mom Does the Work...

Congratulations! Calving is the hard part, and that part is done! The cow will now take care of increasing how much milk the calf gets and when it needs to be increased, and she'll also help teach the calf how to graze and eat grain and obey cow social structure.

A cow's milk production increases over the first two to three months of lactation and then decreases from that peak. The volume produced and the speed at which it decreases depend on the breed, the diet, and whether or not the calf is still nursing.

The three-month peak and then drop-off coincides with the calf being able to make more use of roughage as he reaches that age. Remember, a calf's rumen is not developed at birth, and takes at least 30 days before it even begins to develop the bacteria population required to break down cellulose. The calf will, of course, start nibbling and imitating mom's grazing early on, but this is just the process of getting the rumen primed; he isn't really getting anything out of it.

Parent-raised babies are almost always thriftier (healthy and an "easy keeper") and better nourished and grow a little better. There is just an advantage to getting a meal or snack any time you want one.

Bottle Raising a Calf

If bottle- or bucket-raising a calf, the first thing to do is make sure it has had colostrum. I know I sound like a broken record, but the importance of that first meal of colostrum cannot be overstated, and there is only a short window that it can be absorbed and do any good.

If you have no idea if your bottle calf has had colostrum, consult with your vet right away. There are blood tests that can be done to see what the blood plasma concentration of immunoglobulins (IgGs) is, and that can inform you what sort of battle you will be fighting.

Checklist

- Bottle
- Nipple
  Small calves may not be able to use the larger, heavier rubber nipples that are generally sold with calf bottles. In this case, a lamb nipple will work for the first few days, and then once the calf is nursing well, you can switch to a larger one for a larger bottle. There are lamb nipples that will fit over a plastic soda or water bottle, which should be easily available.
- Milk replacer
  A species-specific milk replacer powder is essential.
- A way to warmup the milk
  Milk replacer should be warm when fed to the calf. It doesn't need to be hot or at a specific temperature, but cold milk replacer is not as palatable initially, and they might not want to drink as much. After the calf is on the bottle well, it isn't as much of a concern.
- Patience

Feeding the Calf

When starting a calf on the bottle, it may take him a little while to catch on. He's not dumb. Especially if he had a chance to nurse from the cow, all of a sudden this rubber nipple thing appears, and it tastes and feels weird. And the milk replacer definitely does not taste like what mama used to make. Be patient. Once he gets the idea that this new stuff fills his empty tummy, he's going to feed enthusiastically.

Make sure to keep his head in the nursing position. If you've ever seen a calf nurse, or any baby animal for that matter, their head and neck are extended downward and the chin juts up so they can latch on to the nipple. This position allows the esophageal groove to close, and the milk bypasses the rumen and goes straight to the abomasum, or true stomach, where it can be digested. Keeping the head in the nursing position will also help keep him from accidentally aspirating (breathing) the milk, which can lead to pneumonia.

Offer an amount based on the recommendations on the package of milk replacer. They will usually recommend an amount based on a percentage of the calf's weight, usually 10–12%. If, once they are nursing well, they seem to still be extremely hungry after a bottle, you can up the amount a bit. Just don't go too far, too fast, or you can cause digestive upset, as their system tries to handle the larger amount.

To get the calf's weight, grab your bathroom scale, pick up the calf and step on. Step off, and subtract your weight from the total weight with the calf. This will give you a close enough weight to work from. You will more than likely have to have someone give you a hand with this. It's next to impossible to hold the calf and peer down around it to read the scale numbers.

Keep the calf warm and dry. In the first couple of weeks, a calf isn't able to regulate his own body temperature very-well, so keeping them out of temperature extremes is important.

If you can feed your calf four to six times a day, at least in the first few days, he will do better. Spacing out the feedings will help his stomach adjust and not fill it too full. After he's nursing well, you can reduce the number of feedings per day. Personally, I try to keep it no fewer than three, just to keep from feeding too much at one time.

As the calf grows, you will need to adjust this amount, and, ultimately, he will get too large for you to pick up and carry on the scale. By then you will have an eye for how fast he's gaining and be able to adjust feeding accordingly.

Whatever schedule you choose, be consistent. Don't feed at 7 a.m. one morning and 10 a.m. the next. The calf is dependent on you for everything, and if he's not sure when his next meal is arriving, it can be stressful. Some variability is normal and expected, but for the next four to six weeks, your schedule should revolve around the calf as much as possible.

If you can, stick to one milk replacer until the calf is weaned. There is always some variability between brands of milk replacer in taste and composition. If that's not possible, for whatever reason, try to mix a little of the old formula with the new to help transition between the two.

Hay and concentrates can begin to be offered in small amounts after the first week or so. While calves don't get much out of them nutritionally, it's important for rumen development and the creation of a healthy microflora population. Offer a small amount of a good calf starter. Starters are designed to be highly

Figuring the Amount to Offer

Once you have the calf's weight in pounds, multiply that by ounces. Take the percentage you want to feed, and multiply that by the weight in ounces. That gives you how many ounces to feed per day. Divide that by the number of feedings you plan to give, and there is your amount per feeding.

So:

Calf weighs 60 lbs., 60 x16 = 960 ounces.

960 ounces x.12 (or 12% of 960) = 115.2 ounces.

115 ounces is the total the calf needs for the day.

If you plan to give four feedings, that will be 28.75 ounces per feeding. (Round that up to 29 oz. Nobody needs to spend the mental energy to measure ¾ of an ounce.)

Metric equivalent: *27 Kg x .12 = 3.25; 3.25/4 = approx. 0.8 Kg per feeding.*

Again, this is a guideline, just to give you a jumping off point.

palatable, and they often contain dried milk products to help encourage the calf to sample. They smell really good to us, too.

A Word about Baby Poop

Normal baby cow poop ranges in color from black and tarry-looking meconium to bright yellow and toothpasty to peanut buttery looking. All these are normal. What is not normal and is a cause for concern is pale, watery stools; bloody stools; or no stools.

Calf scours (diarrhea) is a common ailment, especially in bottle calves, or calves that have not gotten adequate colostrum.

Calf scours can turn fatal very quickly due to dehydration. It won't take long for the calf to lose a critical amount of fluid, and once they get very dehydrated it's hard for them to recover. Calf scours require veterinary attention quickly.

Behavior

Bottle calves really are adorable with their milk slobber faces and the eager way they anticipate your arrival with the daily bottles. It's pretty easy to think they really love you.

Don't fall for it.

One of the potentially most dangerous types of livestock is a bottle calf that has lost respect for humans.

It's cute when they head butt your knees wanting more milk when they weigh a hundred pounds. It definitely isn't cute when they weigh a thousand.

Don't tolerate any head butting, kicking, or pushiness. Cattle are not naturally aggressive, but they will constantly test boundaries to see where their place in the herd hierarchy is. And your answer has always got to be, "Right below the humans, little dude."

I'm not saying you have to be mean to them—far from it. A sharp word or a slap on the shoulder or on the nose is sufficient to get the message across, as long as it's consistently applied. One person can't be the disciplinarian and everyone else in the family let the calf do whatever it wants. That's not fair to the calf. Anyone who can't get on board with enforcing order shouldn't be allowed to feed the calf.

And any male calf that is bottle raised should be castrated. Bottle-raised bulls are simply too dangerous once they begin to feel the rush of those hormones.

Weaning from the Bottle

Any weanling must have access to high-quality feeds at weaning, and it's critical for a bottle calf that will likely be weaned earlier than his mother-raised peers. If he does not get a high-protein feed, designed for early weaned calves, he may not thrive.

If you have given him hay and calf starter as he was bottle-raised, the process will be much easier.

In mother-raised calves, her normal milk production will begin tapering off at about three months, and the calf will start eating more and more pasture, hay, and grain to compensate.

When weaning your bottle calf, you can accomplish the same thing by reducing the amount in the bottle at each feeding and then by removing one bottle per week.

The calf may not appreciate this and will let you know about it. This may also be where inappropriate head butting will also increase. Stick to your guns, and he will adjust quickly.

Weaning from Mom

At some point, the mother-raised calf will need to be weaned from the cow.

Weaning is the most stressful time in the calf's life. Even if he is no longer receiving the bulk of his nutrition from her, he still depends on her for social interaction and security.

Why bother weaning if her milk production is decreasing? Continuing to lactate, even if the calf is not getting the bulk of his nutrition from the cow, can have an adverse effect on her body condition, and if she's bred back (that is, if she's been rebred and pregnant again) this will come at her expense and that of her next calf.

Sometimes you won't be able to separate the mom from the calf and will have no choice but to let her naturally wean him. In this case, make sure they are both being fed at a level that will keep their body condition up, and be generous with your expectations as far as the cow breeding back is concerned.

When to Wean

Most producers try to wean the calf between five and nine months. If the cow is not holding condition well, wean on the earlier side. If both are doing well and on good pasture, you can wait longer. The older the calf, the more he's already used to forage and the less he depends on his mother.

Historically, weaning used to be accomplished without consideration to the stress on the cow or calf. Calves were loaded onto trailers and taken away to feedlots or sale barns, and cows were left to bawl and pace. Calves weaned in this fashion are subjected to more stress and are at higher risk for shipping pneumonia and scours, and even if they do not get sick, the stress will cause them to stall in gaining weight.

Low-stress weaning has gained a lot of ground in recent years. For commercial producers, it helps reduce the cost of treating sick calves, and as the bottom line depends on pounds of beef marketed at a certain time, anything keeping the calves gaining steadily is desirable.

But for those of us with a small herd, low-stress weaning gives us the chance to do better by our calves. There are several methods of low-stress weaning. One involves removing one cow at a time from the herd and moving her to a different paddock or pasture. Usually beginning with the oldest calf's mother, every few days another cow or couple of cows are removed. The calves are left with their peers, so their social structure is still intact. Nutritionally, they don't need mom, and while they may call out a few times, they adjust pretty rapidly. After a time, the cows are all removed, and the calves are still together. This is a bit more labor-intensive as a method of weaning, but it can work well.

A similar method of weaning is called "fenceline weaning." This is exactly how it sounds. The calves and cows are separated into adjacent pastures or paddocks. They are still able to see and talk with one another, but the calf is unable to nurse.

At first, the cows will hang out by the fence near the calves, but eventually they will start to wander off for food and water. They can return whenever they want to but eventually will come back less and less, and everyone adjusts easily. The calves still have their same buddy group and can see mom whenever she stops by.

I can't stress enough that for fenceline weaning to be successful, the fence between the calf and cow has got to be

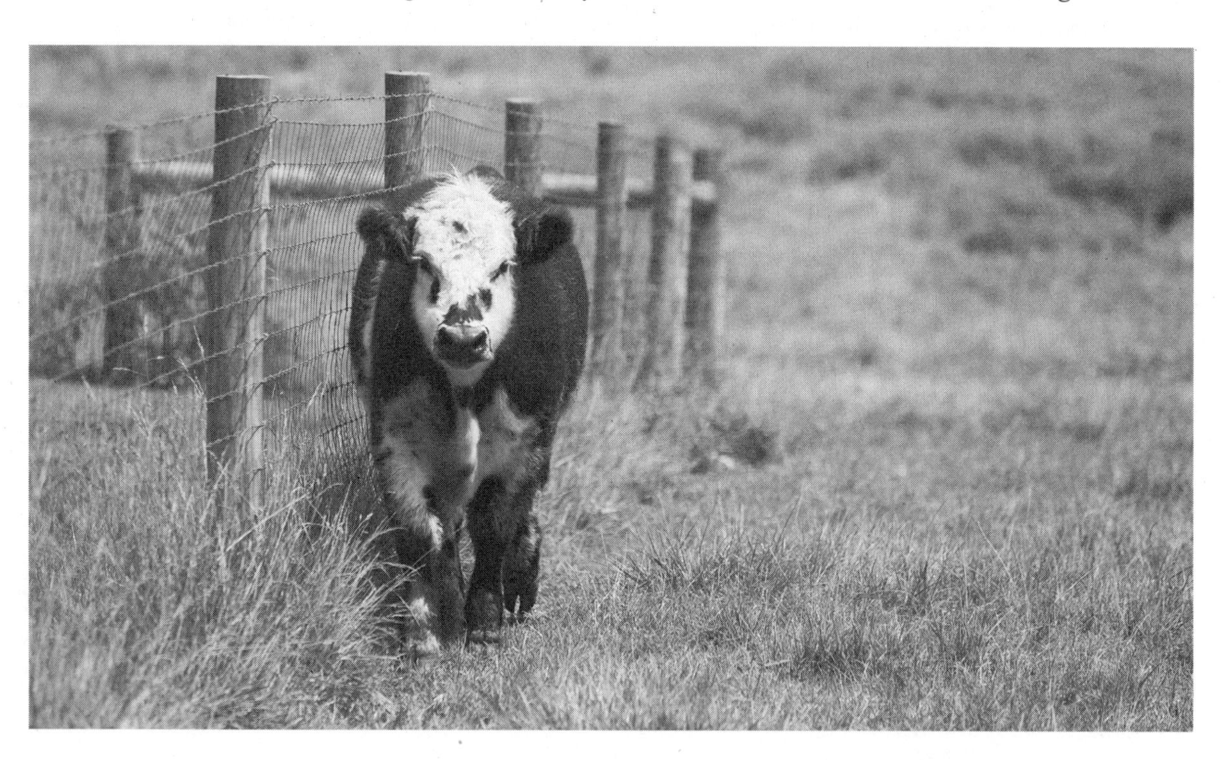

Fenceline calf.
CREDIT: EMILY NYMAN

substantial and physical. Hot wire simply will not work—an extremely motivated calf can slip through or under, willing to ignore the shock. And the potential for the animal to go through the fence, tear it up, and get entangled is too great. A good fence made of cattle panels, corral panels, or sturdy woven wire is a must for fenceline weaning to succeed.

If physically separating the cow and calf isn't an option, there are nose-flap weaners that should be available at farm supply stores or from catalogs. These are little plastic pieces with a sharp edge that fit in a calf's nose. They do not prevent calves from eating or drinking water but the sharp edge will poke the cow and she won't want to nurse. It's not as cruel as it sounds. The weaner flaps are designed to be uncomfortable, not to injure her udder. The down side is you will have to catch the calf to put them in and take them out, and there is always that one cow-calf pair that just doesn't care and she'll still let her calf nurse.

Don't wean in hot weather. Thirty minutes of exertion, by bawling and running the fence, can raise a calf's temperature two degrees. Conversely, cold, wet weather is hard on just-weaned calves as well.

If possible, a green pasture with good shade is the best place to wean a calf. There is no dust, and the calf is in familiar surroundings.

Your cow may have a full, uncomfortable udder for a few days after weaning, depending on her milk production. If your goal is for her to dry up before her next calf is born, don't give in to the temptation to milk her. The pressure of the unmilked udder will cause hormonal signals to kick in, telling her to stop producing milk. Eventually the extra milk will be reabsorbed into her tissues. There is no need to remove it. If you have been milking her all along and sharing with the calf, there is no reason why you cannot continue to do so, but unless you are able to completely empty the udder, over time she will produce less and less.

Buying a Calf for Beef

If your goal is meat for the freezer, instead of breeding and calving a cow, it may be much easier to purchase a calf and raise it to harvest. Home-raised beef is nearly always going to be better quality than store bought, and there is a tremendous sense of pride and satisfaction in growing your own food, whether it's garden produce or meat. Done properly, it can also save you money in the long run.

One of the first expressions you'll hear, as you go looking for a calf to buy, is "bucket calf." Bucket calf refers to a young calf, removed from its mother at one to two days of age. Bucket calves are referred to as such because most of the people who raise them teach them to drink from a bucket rather than a bottle, because the bucket is less work than making up bottles several times a day.

If the calf has just been taken from its mother, it will need to be trained to drink from a bottle or a bucket. Either way, this is not always as easy as it sounds. Initially, the calf may not want to drink something that is not like what mama used to make. The milk replacer tastes strange and comes from a bottle nipple that definitely doesn't feel like mom's udder. Plan to spend a little time, at first, helping them to get the hang of it. As long as the calf is healthy, once he's hungry enough to not be picky, he will catch on pretty quickly.

Switching to a bucket can be a bit harder, as they may not initially understand how to drink from the bucket. If the calf will suckle well, get some milk replacer on your fingers and gradually work your hand and his mouth into the milk bucket. Eventually he'll figure out how it works, and once he realizes it makes him feel full, he'll be on board with the process.

Either bucket or bottle is fine, but the bottle does allow the calf to hold his head in the more natural nursing position.

Considerations for Bringing Home a Bucket Calf

Facilities

Mother cows are very good at finding their calves warm places to hunker down and get out of the weather; you will have to take this role with your calf. Make sure your new calf has adequate shelter. This does not have to be an elaborate barn, or a spot in your living room, but it does need to be clean and dry. A three-sided shed bedded down with clean hay or straw is just fine, and if there is a gate that can be used to close the calf in if necessary, that's a bonus.

A 12 foot × 12 foot (roughly 3.5 m × 3.5 m) pen is a good starter size for the calf. That translates to 144 square feet (about 12 m^2) and should give him ample room to move around. If you are planning to keep him in the pen long term, make sure it's easy for you to get in and clean out the pen with a tractor or loader, otherwise you are looking at a lot of pitchfork time.

If you have the pen set up inside a barn, make sure there are no electrical cords or anything dangerous for him to chew on. A calf that gets to eat only a couple of times a day is going to get bored and want to chew or suck on anything it can get hold of.

Hot wire can be used for fencing, but it is probably not appropriate for a very young calf that you have just brought home. He's confused, doesn't know where he is, and needs to settle in before he's exposed to electric fence. A solid fence is best starting out, and by solid I mean either a sturdy panel or post and wood that he can easily see and that won't give in to pushing. Once he's used to his new home, and if you plan to use hot wire elsewhere on your farm, you can run a string along the existing fence, and let him figure it out. That way if the sudden shock startles him, he's still contained and won't panic and run through the opposite side.

Where to Find Your Calf

One of the most common places to purchase calves is the local sale barn, but there are several cautions with buying calves from there, especially very young ones.

Calves may have started out healthy when they left the farm, but once at the sale barn they are exposed to and mixed with other animals and therefore potentially exposed to a variety of diseases.

Sale barn staff will not be able to tell you anything about the individual calves, either, so it's difficult to ensure that any of the calves got adequate colostrum soon after birth.

Young calves at the sale barn are also experiencing extreme stress at being separated from their mothers. Stress will lower their immune response, and they will become more susceptible to bacteria and diseases.

Purchasing directly from a local breeder might be a better option, and a better chance for a healthy calf. The breeder can tell you whether or not the calf got to nurse from its mother and will know the calf's history and potential better.

However, a breeder might not want to sell a very young calf, because then what is he going to do with a cow with a lot of milk and no calf? The breeder might be more willing to sell you the calf closer to weaning time. This can be a great option; the calf has been raised on his own mother's milk instead of replacer and will be over the hurdles as far as challenges to his immune system go.

If you do wind up with a bucket (or bottle) calf, plan to feed it milk replacer for a minimum of a month and well into the second month. The calf's rumen will not be functioning for the first 30 days, and it will take him some time to begin eating solid food at a rate high enough to keep him growing well. The closer you can get to three months before trying to wean, the better.

Signs of a Healthy Calf

A healthy calf is bright eyed, curious, active, and shiny coated. When a calf that feels good gets up, it will (unless it was startled and got up abruptly) take a second or two for a good stretch and then move along. Normally a healthy calf will sleep curled up, with its feet tucked under and head curled back around. On occasion, a healthy calf will sleep flat out on his side, but it's unusual enough that it bears a second glance.

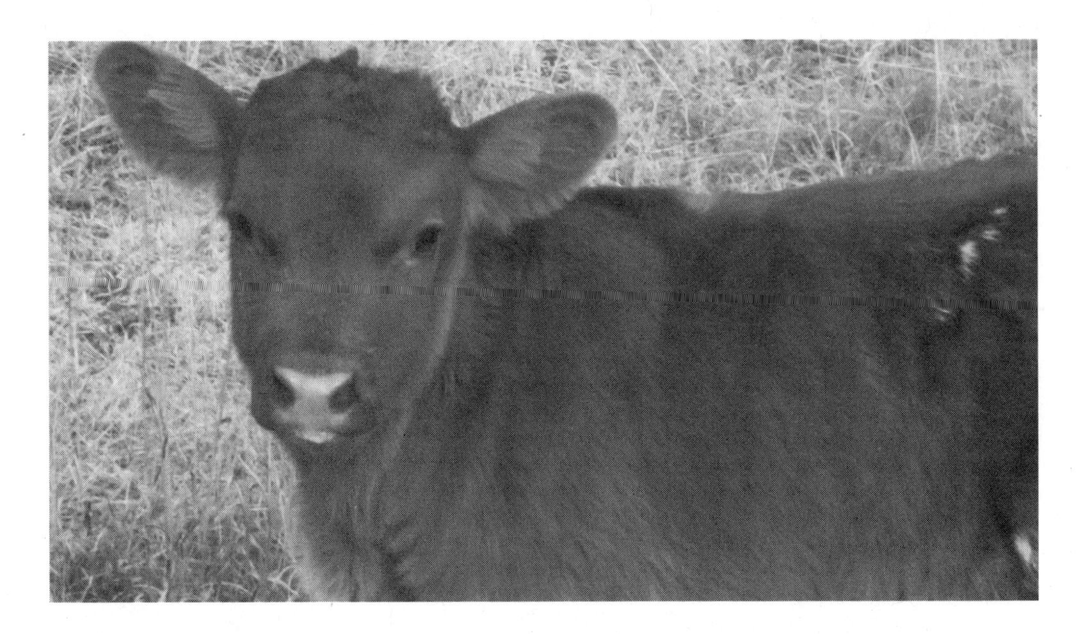

Alert calf.

When you approach a healthy calf, it will be alert and aware of your presence. Depending on how shy he is he may run back to mama or cautiously approach you. On a warm day, a calf may breathe rapidly, but the breath should not be labored.

On the flip side, a calf that does not feel well will have a dull, listless appearance. He may not stretch when he gets up, because he doesn't feel well and is apathetic about everything going on around him. Watch for signs of bloat—if the calf's side is swollen up larger than normal, it's cause for concern. Watch the rump for signs of scours. An infected calf will invariably get loose stool on his tail, and smear it all over his rump. A calf with a clean rump is usually doing okay. Watch the nose and eyes for signs of discharge. The tear ducts and nasal passages are closely linked, and if the calf has a cold, he may have nasal discharge combined with eye boogers. And, if a normally active, hungry calf suddenly has no desire to drink his bottle or eat the grain you offer, it's a cue that something serious is going on.

CHAPTER 9

Cattle Health

THE OLD ADAGE about shutting the barn door after the horse has gotten out is often instructive, including as it applies to the health of your cattle.

Focusing on preventative care will go a lot further than reacting when an animal gets sick. Even then, if one does get sick, your problem may not be as serious, because you did not start out behind the eight ball.

OK, enough metaphors.

A cow cannot have an effective immune system if her nutritional needs are not being met. The first and foremost thing a conscientious cow owner should do is take a good look at diet and body condition. If your cows are in good flesh (have ample muscle and fat) and are shiny and bright eyed, their immune systems are functioning at a higher level than a cow that is not in good condition.

Sanitation is also important. Fresh air and sunshine do a lot for a cow's well-being, and they are also good disinfectants.

Sanitation doesn't have to mean disinfecting and scrubbing everything with chemicals. Keeping manure cleaned out of sheds, birthing areas, and winter feeding pens helps to keep parasites and germs from building up to a level that can challenge even a healthy immune system. (This is where you will come to love that old tractor!) Good old soap and water and sunlight work great for cleaning tanks, feed bunks, and all sorts of equipment—and they don't cost much.

Don't overstock pens and pastures. When given the opportunity, cattle are pretty good about not wanting to eat where they defecate. If there are too many cows for the size of their pasture, they can't help but come into contact with feces. Rotational grazing methods can help keep both your pasture and your cows healthy.

Parasite problems will also be reduced with good management. Depending on the parasite and the life cycle, rotating animals off of pastures for a time can help break up the cycle and reduce their exposure to parasite eggs and larvae.

The more you are able to maintain a closed herd and minimize bringing animals in and out frequently, the better chance you have of not introducing something to your established group of cows.

When adding a new cow to your herd, especially if she comes from an unknown source, quarantine her away from the rest of the herd for two to four weeks. This gives her a chance to settle in and gives you a chance to observe her for any signs of illness, catching it before the rest of your herd are exposed to her. It doesn't have to be complete lockdown, but keep her from having nose contact with the rest of your cows if possible and from defecating where they will graze.

Minimize stress whenever possible. One of the biggest stressors for cattle is being handled, especially if they are not used to it happening on a regular basis. Even the cow that gets milked daily benefits from a low-stress environment.

Stress hinders normal immune system functioning. When an animal experiences stress, the flood of cortisol inhibits the normal immune response and antibody production. This is why shipping animals long distances is problematic. The stress of travel, combined with being exposed to other cattle and whatever *they* have been exposed to, is a recipe for illness.

Don't do procedures such as castration at weaning, which is one of the most stressful times in a calf's life. Either do this early on, while he is still nursing from mom, or a couple of weeks after he's settled down from weaning. And of course, the earlier the bull calf gets castrated, the easier it is on both him and you.

Castration

Castration is typically done in one of two ways. Either a sharp scalpel is used to open the scrotum and the testicles are manually removed, or a special rubber band is applied with a special tool.

I've had decent luck using the banding tool on very young animals. There seems to be little pain, and it doesn't take long for the testicles to wither and fall off. The downside is that it can be hard to find both testicles in a very young animal, and you sure don't want to remove just one. Larger animals with more developed testicles will have more pain when banded, and it will take longer for the testicles to wither and fall off.

Using a scalpel is quicker and heals faster, but unless you've done something like this before, have a vet or an experienced cattle person show you the first few times.

My honest preference is to let the vet do it, especially if the calf gets some size to him before it's done. It's an additional expense, but with one or two calves it might be worth it for the expertise. A vet can also give an injection of painkillers to help both you and the calf feel better faster.

If you elect not to castrate, the bull calf will reach puberty before you know it, and then you have a whole other set of bad behaviors to potentially worry about.

Let your cows get accustomed to any facilities you plan to use well before they are first needed. Our chute is positioned right on the way to the water tank, where they have to pass by multiple times per day. Our rotational grazing system means they will come into that lot from every angle and path possible, and our load out chute is near one of the common areas as well. We move them into the chute in the same direction that they use to go to the water. All this means that on any day they have to go into the chute, not all that much is different from their usual routines.

Behavior and Appearance of Healthy Cattle

We've talked about the appearance of healthy cattle before, but it doesn't hurt to repeat it.

One of the best indicators of healthy cattle is a shiny coat. It's more than just aesthetics, a shiny coat means the cow's nutritional needs are being met. If there is not adequate protein directly available from the diet, or being manufactured by the rumen, the coat will appear dull. Protein is an essential building block for the hair coat, and if the coat is dull and wiry looking, you can bet either the diet isn't quite right or there is a parasite load interfering with absorption of nutrients.

Healthy cattle are active. They move around to graze, get water, and find a comfortable spot to chew their cud. They also congregate together, and tend to move as a herd when grazing.

By contrast, cattle that aren't feeling well will often hang out by themselves and not move around with the herd. They may have dull eyes and a dull haircoat and be lying down when the rest of the herd is grazing.

Cattle typically lie down and curl their front legs under their sternum and will often curl their head around to rest their head on their shoulder in a position that looks anything but comfortable to us. What they hardly ever do, unless they are sick, is lie flat out on their sides. Anytime you see that, it's a cue to check things out.

In warmer weather, cattle may have a nasal discharge, as they breathe more rapidly to cool off. Normal nasal discharge will be clear; abnormal will be yellowish and look like what we get with a bad cold. They may also have discharge from the eyes, as the sinuses and tear ducts are linked. A mild case might be something the cow can shake off herself; more severe might need a visit from the vet.

Always contact your vet if you have health concerns, but it's up to you to learn to recognize problems.

Vets would much rather work with you to come up with a preventative program than wait until your animals are sick. Yes, vets charge money for their services and make their living from it, but I've never met one yet who wouldn't 100 times rather help prevent animal illness instead of treat it.

One thing to keep handy is a simple thermometer. Being able to take a cow's or calf's temperature can clue you in to how serious a problem might be. A fever generally means a call to the vet is in order, and the more data you can give your vet, the better he or she will be able to help you.

A cow's temperature is taken by inserting a thermometer into the rectum. An inexpensive digital baby thermometer works great, and usually the ends are flexible. Normal temperature is 101, but don't panic at a half a degree either way, depending on weather and activity level. For a calf, anything over 102 might call for action.

Antibiotics

Antibiotics as we know them today are a relatively modern thing, not widely formulated or used before WWII. I'm not even going to pretend to condone or defend their widespread use in the agriculture industry. We are all keenly aware of the issues with antibiotic resistance and the continuous adaptability of bacteria.

But! A sick animal should receive treatment. End of discussion. It's simply not ethical to allow an animal to be sick and miserable if you can help. There are enough things that are out of our control; let's take care of what is within our power to help.

Even if that means antibiotics. Using antibiotics at the recommendation of your vet to treat a specific problem can save you time and heartache down the road. It can shorten the duration of illness, lessen its severity, and keep the animal from suffering as much.

There is a mile of difference between using antibiotics to treat an animal in your care that is ill, and using antibiotics as growth promoters or to compensate for poor management.

Keep the use of antibiotics as a tool in your tool box, to be used properly and judiciously. Good management can make sure it's a tool of last resort.

And a final note: always be aware of, and follow strictly, the withdrawal times listed on the labels.

Immunity and Vaccinations

There are two basic types of immunity: passive and active.

Passive immunity is what happens when a calf receives antibodies in his mother's colostrum. They are absorbed through the lining of the intestine into the bloodstream and provide him, for a short time, with the same antibody protection the cow has. Without that, the calf has no antibody response of his own and is vulnerable to any bacteria or immune challenge he will come across in his environment. This is not to say he does not have any immune response whatsoever. His own system will begin fighting off challenges, but without any maternal protection, it is easy for his system to be overwhelmed.

Calves will begin to lose this maternal antibody protection at about eight weeks, which is why most vaccination programs recommend a first round at that age. Trying to give vaccinations earlier than eight weeks can interfere with, or be blocked by, the maternal antibodies, and the calf's own immune response will not respond adequately.

Active immunity is the calf's own immune response. It is generated by exposure to pathogens or by vaccination, which triggers the immune response. Healthy animals are able to mount a strong immune response and defend themselves against pathogens, as long as they are not subject to an overwhelming load of bacteria or virus.

Vaccination provides an enhanced immune response to specific pathogens. When the vaccination occurs, the animal's immune system mounts a response to the deactivated or killed pathogen. The system develops a "memory," enabling the animal to mount a defense faster than if it were being exposed for the first time. With limited immunity, the invading organism multiplies rapidly and the result can be illness or death.

Vaccination against a disease does not mean the calf will never get the disease if exposed to it. It just means that the severity will hopefully be lessened and the recovery much faster.

I completely understand not wanting to give your cow and calf a bunch of injections if they aren't needed. There are a number of diseases that vaccines are available for. Depending on where you live, some may not be necessary in your area. But some are highly recommended: diseases such as Leptospirosis can be transmitted by wildlife, and Clostridial bacteria are prevalent in the soil. Vaccination can help prevent both of these diseases. Consult with your vet for more information on what's best for your farm.

Most vaccines are relatively perishable and need to be stored in a refrigerator, at around 35–45°F (2–7°C). Temperatures too warm or too cold can inactivate and damage the vaccine and render it less effective. Don't insert a used needle into the vaccine bottle, and try to keep everything clean during the vaccination process. Syringes can be cleaned with warm water and reused.

Common Health Problems in Cattle

The following discussion of health problems that cattle can experience is by no means exhaustive. I've chosen to focus on the ones that you will be most likely to run into and the ones that can best be prevented with good management.

Rather than redundantly ending each paragraph with the advice to always consult with your veterinarian, I'll just preface the entire section with the advice that, in any situation when an animal is sick or you have questions about vaccines or treatment, always consult with your veterinarian.

Health Problems for Calves

Scours

Scours is characterized by watery, profuse, foul-smelling diarrhea that can lead to dehydration, and if it is not treated it can quickly become fatal.

Scours is a common problem in young calves in the first two to four weeks of life, especially if they did not get an adequate meal of colostrum within the first eight hours of life.

Scours can also be caused or made worse by an unclean environment. If the cow is lying down in dirty bedding or in mud, and her udder is dirty, when the calf nurses it will ingest bacteria and develop scours. Keep calf housing clean and dry.

There are several vaccines available that can be given to pregnant cows at various stages of gestation. These can help boost the cows' immunity, and thereby the quality of protection in the colostrum, but the colostrum may or may not contain antibodies for a specific bacteria that can cause diarrhea.

Situations that cause stress, such as a difficult delivery, cold and wet weather, crowding, and uncleanliness, can all contribute to the onset and severity of scours, even in otherwise healthy animals.

Navel Ill

Navel ill is a catch-all term that can describe several conditions, all arising from bacterial contamination of the umbilical cord and stump soon after calving. After birth, when the navel cord breaks, the blood vessels that supplied the calf during gestation will contract and dry up, but for a time until the cord stump dries, bacterial contamination can enter the bloodstream. If the contamination settles in the joints it can cause severe joint infections. If it stays local to the umbilicus, it can cause an abscess and an umbilical infection. This is, fortunately, easier to treat than the joint infections.

E. Coli is also a common bacteria that can enter the bloodstream through the navel and cause life threatening infections, scours, and death. Even if the calf survives, it may never thrive.

The best defense against navel ill is to make sure calves are born into a clean environment, and treat the navel cord soon after birth with a 7% iodine solution. This will not only help kill any bacteria but will also help dry up the stump, shutting off access for bacteria.

Pneumonia

Pneumonia is probably the second biggest killer of young calves, right after scours. The bacteria and viruses that cause pneumonia can be lurking in the environment, and if stress weakens the calf's immune system, they can strike.

A calf with pneumonia will have a temperature of 103–104°F (39.5–40°C) or higher. He will experience labored breathing, coughing, or runny nose, may not want to eat or drink, and will stand with a hunched appearance.

If mild, or caught early, pneumonia can be treated with antibiotics, usually over a course of several days. Care will need to be taken to keep the calf in a warm, dry environment until treatment is complete, as any stress will make the condition worse and the treatment less effective.

Health Problems for Cows

Calves can also experience any of these issues.

Ringworm

Ringworm is a fungus, not a worm. The name comes from the round patches of lost hair that characterize the problem. Ringworm can be treated with specially medicated shampoos and antifungals to prevent spread to other animals, and to humans. Left untreated, ringworm will usually clear up on its own but may become quite severe and uncomfortable before it does.

Pinkeye

Pinkeye is a contagious bacterial infection of the eye, exhibited by watery eye discharge, redness and swelling of the eye, sensitivity to sunlight, and keeping eyes closed.

It is spread by face flies and can rapidly spread throughout a herd. If severe, or left untreated, it can cause lesions on the cornea, and the eye can become permanently damaged.

Fortunately, it responds well to treatment. There are several ointments and sprays that can be put into the eye. Unfortunately, this requires catching the animal and treating multiple times. Many producers prefer to just give an antibiotic injection.

Blackleg

Blackleg is one of a suite of Clostridial diseases that are caused by bacteria living in the soil. These bacteria are anaerobic, meaning they thrive in conditions that are not exposed to air, such as inside the body. Tetanus is a clostridial disease. While clostridia cannot be passed from animal to animal, if the spores are present on the farm, which they likely are, multiple animals may be infected. Unfortunately, often the first sign of Clostridial disease is a dead cow, as the bacteria produces toxins rapidly.

Vaccines are readily available. A "7 way" vaccine contains vaccine for all seven of the clostridial strains, and an "8 way" covers all those plus tetanus.

Brucellosis

Brucellosis is a highly contagious bacterial disease, causing abortion in cattle and other ruminants. Also called Bang's disease, it can also affect humans. Stopping the spread of brucellosis, in particular, was one of the major reasons milk pasteurization requirements were initiated. It causes undulant fever in humans because of the severe, intermittent fever that goes with human infection.

Brucellosis is spread by contact with infected animals, with highly infectious afterbirth, or with vaginal secretions and fluids after a cow has aborted. (*Always* wear OB sleeves or rubber gloves when handling materials and tissue from aborted fetuses.) Other animals coming in contact with the infected placental membranes or fluids can also contract the disease.

It can spread from cattle to ruminant wildlife such as bison, elk, and deer, and can also be transmitted from native animals to cattle.

In 1954, a Brucellosis Eradication Program was begun in the United States. This involved vaccinating calves, testing herds, and sending infected animals to slaughter. Over the years, the rate of infection dropped from 124,000 affected herds, to 700 in 1992, and at the time of this writing, all 50 US states are brucellosis free, as is Canada.

Because of the seriousness of this disease and it's potential for human infection, brucellosis is considered a disease reportable to the government. Populations of wild animals are also monitored to prevent the disease being spread to domestic animals, resulting in a state losing its brucellosis-free status.

There is a vaccine, but it must be given by a licensed veterinarian, who will then put a metal brucellosis tag (often called a Bang's tag) in the animal's ear so there is an official record of its vaccination. Antibodies will be present in a vaccinated animal, so a record of the vaccination is vital to prevent unnecessary reporting of the disease. If you live in an area with a high concentration of elk, bison, or deer, discuss vaccination strategies with your veterinarian.

Johne's Disease

Johne's (pronounced yoh-nees) is a disease that affects ruminants, caused by the bacteria *Mycobacterium avium paratuberculosis*, or MAP. This bacteria attacks the small intestine and, as the tissues try to mount an immune response, the intestine thickens, leading to poor nutrient absorption. Progressive weight loss and diarrhea occur, and ultimately death. There is no cure, and while a vaccine has been developed, there is some question about how effective it is. It can also interfere with TB test results.

Sheep and goats and beef cattle, can be affected, but it is of special concern in the dairy industry. The USDA estimates that up to 68% of the dairy herds in the US will have at least one cow test positive for Johne's.[4]

Part of the trouble with controlling Johne's is that the disease is very slow in its progression, so animals may be shedding the bacteria and not show any symptoms. Johne's is spread primarily by contact with bacteria shed in the feces. The bacteria can then infect the soil and water and remain viable for a year or more. A cow could pick up the bacteria as a calf and not show any signs or symptoms for years. There is also evidence that it can be passed in utero, if the cow is in the later stages of the disease, and it can also be passed in milk from infected mothers. Because of the slow progression of Johne's, cattle less than 2 years of age will likely not show any clinical signs even if exposed at birth. Older animals exposed to the bacteria for the first time may be somewhat resistant to it, but if the presence of the bacteria is overwhelming, any natural resistance may be overcome.

There are fecal tests and blood tests that can detect the presence of MAP, but they do not work very well to identify subclinical cases, so even if cows that test positive are removed from the herd, some might remain. A third test involves culturing the bacteria, but it is expensive and time consuming.

The best method of controlling Johne's is through biosecurity practices. Buy cows, especially dairy cows, from herds that are Johne's negative, or at least have enough of a testing history to have some idea of their herd status.

Viral Diseases

There are several respiratory problems that cattle can experience. Fortunately, there are vaccines available for the majority of them, so with a good vaccination program and good management, you may never experience them at all.

Infectious Bovine Rhinotracheitis (IBR) is a viral disease that can cause respiratory disease and also abortion in pregnant cattle. One of the most common cattle diseases, it can spread rapidly, especially if cattle are confined closely. Symptoms include a high fever (104°F or higher, 40°C+), inflammation of the nostrils (it is also called "red nose" disease), difficulty breathing, nasal discharge that turns into long, yellowy strings of mucus, and coughing.

Bovine Viral Diarrhea (BVD) is another viral disease that can cause abortion, but also contributes to other illnesses because of its effect on the immune system. Signs of infection also include fever, nasal discharge, loss of appetite, as well as diarrhea. Some cattle may be persistently affected and pass it to their calves in utero, or the fetus may die and become mummified.

Parainfluenza type 3 (PI-3) can be a relatively mild sickness by itself, but it can cause big problems when combined with bacterial infections. It is part of the group of respiratory problems called shipping fever.

Bovine Respiratory Syncytial Virus (BRSV) is another pneumonia-causing virus. It can be hard to detect in bloodwork. It is probably one of the major contributors to pneumonias in calves.

Vaccines exist for all of the above-mentioned viruses, fortunately. Vaccines will list on the label the diseases they are intended to treat, which is why knowing the alphabet soup of letters associated with each disease is important. Many brands of vaccine will cover multiple diseases, which reduces the number of injections you have to give to the cow. Some of the vaccines are modified live vaccines, which basically means they cause a light case of the disease in the animal to trigger its immune response. In the case of the diseases that can cause abortion, the modified live vaccine can actually cause the cow to abort. Do not give those vaccines unless you are 100% sure the cow is not pregnant.

Unfortunately, viral diseases cannot be treated with antibiotics. Should your cow come down with a viral disease, the best you can do for her is provide supportive care, keep her warm and dry and not stressed, and keep your fingers crossed that she recovers.

Bloat

Bloat is a rather benign sounding name for a condition that can be fatal in cattle. Bloat occurs when the cow is not able to eructate, or belch, and gas builds up in the rumen.

As cattle digest and ruminate, they regurgitate and rechew and ingest the contents of the rumen. They also release a lot of gas during this process.

Should the cow not be able to eructate, for whatever reason, the buildup of gas can be so severe that it can quickly become fatal. The rumen presses on the diaphragm and lungs, and eventually the cow will suffocate. Not a pleasant way to go, for sure.

There are two types of bloat, frothy and free gas.

In free gas bloat, there is often a physical obstruction such as a foreign body, tumor, or abscess keeping the gas from being able to be expelled. It can also be caused by posture. A cow cannot eructate when she is lying on her back, so if she falls into a ditch or becomes trapped on her back, she will quickly bloat and die if not corrected. Should a ruminant require surgery, all food should be taken away at least 12 (preferably 24) hours before the surgery so the rumen will be empty and the vet will have time to work.

The second type of bloat, frothy bloat, is more common and also called feedlot bloat or pasture bloat. Frothy bloat occurs when gas becomes trapped in the foam from rapidly digesting feeds such as high-starch concentrates or lush legume pasture.

The foam does not allow the cow to belch and release the gas, and the gas can build up quite rapidly and can be fatal in as little as an hour.

Pasture bloat is caused by the cow suddenly ingesting a lot of rich feed, such as could result from being turned out on alfalfa pasture or placed on a diet that is mostly grain.

The rumen contains one population of microbes for digesting grasses and has different microbes for digesting grains and legumes. When a cow that has been accustomed to hay is suddenly turned out on alfalfa pasture, for example, her microbe population cannot accommodate the sudden change in diet. Cattle on grain-only diets, such as those in feedlots, are prone to bloat, even if they are put on the grain gradually, as the acidic environment created by the rapidly digesting starches leads to foam development in the rumen.

Signs of Bloat

One of the classic signs of bloat is distension of the abdomen, on the left side. Not to be confused with a cow that has a full "grass belly," the distension will extend past the spinous processes and be level with the topline.

The cow will stop eating—if she can't belch anything out, she can't take anything more in. She'll be reluctant to move and will be visibly distressed and anxious. She may pant rapidly, with head and neck extended, trying to get enough air into her lungs to survive. And once she goes down, she's unlikely to survive.

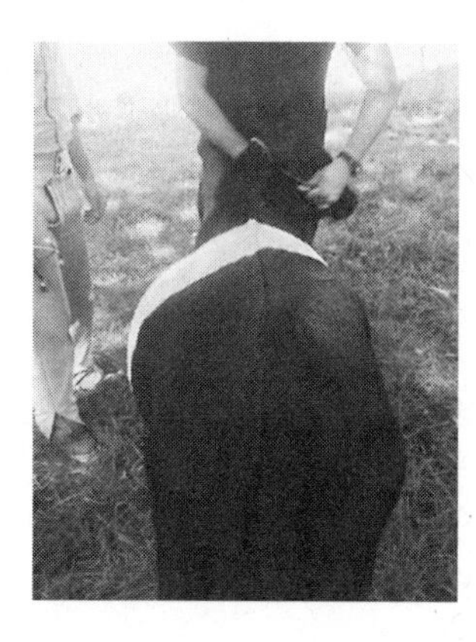

Calf with bloat.
Credit: Stephanie Buchanan

Treatment for Bloat

If you suspect your cow is bloating, get your vet on the phone right away. Treatment for bloat is simple, but it must be done immediately. In severe cases of bloat the vet can use a rumen trochar to poke a hole in the rumen from the outside, and relieve the pressure. This procedure is usually successful but comes with risks (such as peritonitis if rumen contents leak into the abdominal cavity) and should be a last resort.

In a less severe case, or one that is caught early, a tube can be passed through the esophagus to the rumen. In the case of free gas bloat, the relief will be immediate, and you can actually see the animal's distension ease. With frothy bloat, the foam cannot come out through the tube as easily as gas can. An antifoaming agent, such as vegetable oil or mineral oil, can be given via a stomach tube. This will break up the foam and allow the gas to escape.

Prevention of Bloat

Fortunately, bloat is much more easily prevented than treated.

Legume pastures such as alfalfa and clover are great for cows nutritionally; just take care to never turn the cows out when they are hungry. Make sure they have filled up on grass hay prior to turnout, and turn them out for only a short time at first. Or maintain pastures that have grass mixed in with the legumes.

Legumes are richest when they are in the early stage of growth. Once they begin to flower, the risk goes down. Allow the cow's digestive system to adapt to the legumes over a period of a couple of weeks. It will take at least that long for the different microbes to adjust. The same advice applies as well to introducing grains to the diet.

There are other legumes that do not seem to induce bloat as easily as alfalfa and clover. Birdsfoot trefoil, lespedeza, and cowpeas seem to rarely cause bloat, but it is still prudent to introduce cattle to them slowly.

Keep a routine feed schedule also. Allowing the cow to have an empty rumen can disrupt the microbiome.

Parasites

Parasites are an inevitable challenge of working with livestock. It's next to impossible to create an environment with no parasite activity, although good management can certainly reduce the effect they have on your cattle.

There are two types of parasites: external ones, such as lice, flies, and ticks, and internal ones, such as roundworms, coccidia, and flukes. Depending on your geographic area and environment, you may experience problems with many types of parasites or only a few.

Parasites are of concern because of the impact they have on the animal, but they can also have an impact on your bottom line. They can interfere with digestion. They take nutrients away from the host, your cow, causing you to spend money feeding them rather than the animal. Poor nutrient absorption can reduce milk production and reduce conception rate. Parasites can weaken the immune system, making animals more susceptible to disease. And in extreme cases, parasites can lead to anemia, diarrhea, and even death.

There are many species and classes of parasite, but one of the most common ones cattle producers will run across are roundworm (nematodes), most commonly the brown stomach worm, *Ostertagia*. The adult form of this worm grazes the lining of the abomasum, causes fluid loss, and interferes with digestion by affecting the function of the gastric glands in the stomach.

Their life cycle is typical of most internal parasites. The adults produce eggs, which are expelled from the host onto the pasture grass. Larvae hatch from the eggs, molt through several stages until they become infective, and then migrate onto moist grass. As cattle graze, they ingest the infectious larvae, and the life cycle is completed.

Ostertagia can be particularly problematic because they have the ability to enter into an "inhibited" state, which is much like hibernation. This allows them to avoid adverse conditions such as cold winter weather or hot and dry weather, depending on the geographic region. When conditions are more favorable—i.e., when spring weather comes or rain after a period of dry conditions—the larvae will resume growth.

Telltale signs of a heavy *Ostertagia* infestation are "bottle jaw" (an accumulation of fluid around the jaw) and anemia. A rough hair coat, diarrhea, and weight loss are also evident.

Liver flukes are another common parasite in cattle, especially cattle that are grazed in wetland conditions. Flukes require two hosts: cows and snails. Adult flukes are found in the bile ducts of cattle. Eggs are laid in the ducts and expelled in the feces. The larval stage of the fluke infects snails, and from there specific stages of juvenile flukes encyst on aquatic plants. Cattle eat the plants, and the fluke then migrates to the liver.

Coccidia are microscopic protozoa that infect the cells lining the blood vessels in the small intestine. Bloody scours and anemia, and subsequent dehydration, are symptoms of a coccidia infestation. Young animals, between a month and a year of age, are most commonly affected by coccidia, but any age group can be infected. If you observe bloody stools in your cattle, it's best to have a fecal test done to confirm coccidia, as several infectious diseases, such as salmonella and bovine viral diarrhea, also can cause blood in the stool.

Coccidia oocysts (eggs) frequently contaminate feed and water. Susceptibility to coccidia can vary, and other factors such as stress can cause animals to be overwhelmed by a coccidia load.

Keep calving areas clean and pastures well drained to help prevent coccidia, and don't let animals drink from pools of water that have been contaminated by feces.

Fecal egg counts are a test that your veterinarian can perform in his office to give you some sort of idea what the parasite load is. These tests literally measure the number of parasite eggs that are being shed, or excreted, by the host. The test involves collecting a fecal sample, mixing the sample with a reagent, and looking for parasite eggs under the microscope. A large number of fecal eggs in a particular sample is indicative of how many adults are infesting the host. Depending on the life-cycle stage of the parasite, there may or may not be eggs in the fecal sample, although it's unlikely that there would be no parasites shedding at a particular moment. Since fecal tests are easy to do and relatively inexpensive, doing a second test in about two weeks can help confirm the diagnosis.

The most accurate diagnosis of a parasite infestation is a post mortem exam of the affected cow. Hopefully, that won't be something you will have to do.

Strategies to Reduce Parasitism

Parasite activity tends to peak in the spring, when pastures are usually moist with spring rain, decline as the weather becomes hotter and drier, and then have a smaller peak in the fall.

One of the best ways to reduce parasite load is to not overgraze. Normally, cows will not graze close to where they have defecated. But if pastures are overgrazed to the point that they have no choice, parasite infestation is likely to be a greater problem.

Parasites also will travel up only the first few inches of the grass leaf. Cattle prefer to graze the tops of the blades of grass, so by keeping pasture grass over 4 inches tall, they will be less likely to ingest parasite larva as they graze.

Put vulnerable animals on pastures that have not been grazed in the past 12 months. While this may not be practical on the majority of farms, keeping pastures that have not been overgrazed, and using them for young animals or animals that have been stressed for some reason or another, will help reduce the exposure to parasites.

Drain or fence off access to wet areas to reduce exposure to flukes.

Pastures can also be drag harrowed, which has the effect of spreading out clumps of manure and exposing larvae to the elements. This is best done during hotter and drier weather, and then keep animals off pastures for two to three weeks.

Deworming

There are several products that are available for deworming cattle. Dewormers are divided into classes of drug type by the deworming agent, and each class is effective on different parasites. This is why it's important to have an idea of what parasite you are actually experiencing trouble with, and go after that one accordingly.

All medications are dosed by body weight, and dewormers are no different. While it's not necessary to have a precise weight, a close estimate is helpful. If taking your animal to a scale isn't practical, there are weight tapes available from livestock supply companies that will get close; also there are formulas by which you can measure your animal and get a close estimate as well. Underdosing dewormers doesn't do an effective job and may contribute to dewormer resistance. Most deworming products are relatively safe if you overdose slightly, but it's not economical, and too much of an overdose can be harmful.

It's also important not to administer dewormers haphazardly. Resistance to dewormers is an inevitable effect of natural mutations in the parasites. Some parasites will have a natural ability to resist the dewormer. All of the non-resistant parasites will be killed, and guess what happens. The only ones left are the ones that the drug doesn't work on.

Previously, advice on deworming had producers deworming regularly, and deworming all the animals in the herd, whether or not there was an actual problem. This led to the rapid increase of resistant populations of worms.

Research has shown that in a herd, only a percentage of the animals are shedding large amounts of the parasite. Individual fecal tests can identify those animals, and by targeting your deworming efforts to those animals, parasite load can be dramatically decreased.

Cattle are also able to mount a natural immunity to parasites. A low exposure to a parasite can trigger the immune system response, and a healthy cow on good nutrition can manage to keep ahead of a problem.

A new concept that has emerged in recent years around the subject of dewormer resistance involves what is known as "refugia." This involves deworming a part of a cattle herd and not deworming a small percentage. The theory behind this is that by deworming everyone, only the parasites that are susceptible are killed, and the ones that are not susceptible remain to...yep—shed resistant eggs, and the number of resistant parasites increases exponentially. By leaving some animals shedding non-resistant parasites, the population of resistant parasites in the herd overall is diluted, and it will take a longer time for the entire group to be resistant to the dewormer.

External Parasites

External parasite are a problem not only for the toll they take on the cow herself, but they can also be potential vectors for transmission of disease. Flies that bite and suck blood will travel from cow to cow and can pass blood-borne disease as they do.

Horn flies are small black flies that tend to congregate around the horns of cattle or along the back and sides and the poll area of cattle without horns. They bite and suck blood, taking up to 20 meals a day. They affect the cows primarily by the blood they take, but, also, a heavy fly problem can make the cattle so uncomfortable that they aren't able to graze and eat as much as they normally would.

Stable flies are larger than horn flies, and tend to congregate on the legs and under the bellies of cattle. Their bite is more painful than that of the horn fly, causing cattle to stomp, bunch up to swat each other's flies, or stand in water to avoid getting bitten. Stable flies will bite and feed until they are full, resting in shaded areas to digest their blood meal.

Black horse flies may get their name from their favored equine meal, but they have no problem biting cattle either. Their mouth parts are huge, and their bite is very painful.

Warble flies are often called grubs. These flies lay eggs that hatch and penetrate the skin, generally on the legs, where they migrate through the connective tissue to the esophagus. Once there, they travel back to the skin, and cause swellings called "warbles." When a warble is destroyed by pressure, the larvae cause large purulent swellings, and when flies emerge they leave holes in the skin. While the larvae migrate, they can damage the meat tissue, creating tunnels that can fill with a greenish-yellow gelatinous mass, called "butcher's jelly," that makes the meat inedible.

Lice are another external parasite. There are two types: biting and sucking lice. Lice tend to favor cool, damp weather, and will often gravitate toward an animal that might already have a vulnerable immune system for some reason or other. Older animals will develop immunity over time, hence lice can be a bigger problem for young animals that have not had a chance to develop immunity. Lice cause severe itching and hair loss, and if the infestation is great enough, it can cause anemia.

Control of external parasites can be managed by providing insecticide rubs for cattle to use while in pasture. There are dust bags that can be loaded with an insecticide dust, as well as oilers that are soaked with an insecticide containing oil. Cattle quickly learn that they can get relief from the insects by using the bag or oiler. Lice may require treatment with a topical insecticide that will need to be repeated, as nothing is effective on the lice eggs. A single tame cow may benefit from fly sprays, but those are not likely practical in a herd out on pasture.

Giving an Injection

Whenever possible, have the cow restrained to give an injection. Given correctly, an injection can be done before the cow even knows what happened, but if she does figure it out, she might object. Restraint can be having her head tied, or it can be having the cow in a chute.

There are three types of injections: intravenous (IV), subcutaneous (SubQ), and intramuscular (IM). Each type of injection allows the body to absorb the drug in a different way. Each drug is formulated to work in a certain way, and the method of delivery into the body will make sure the drug functions like it should.

It is highly unlikely that you will ever need to give a drug IV; most drugs that work directly in the bloodstream should be given by a veterinarian. Putting a drug directly into the bloodstream means it will act very quickly, and injecting drugs IV that are not designed to work that way can produce very bad results and can possibly even kill the animal.

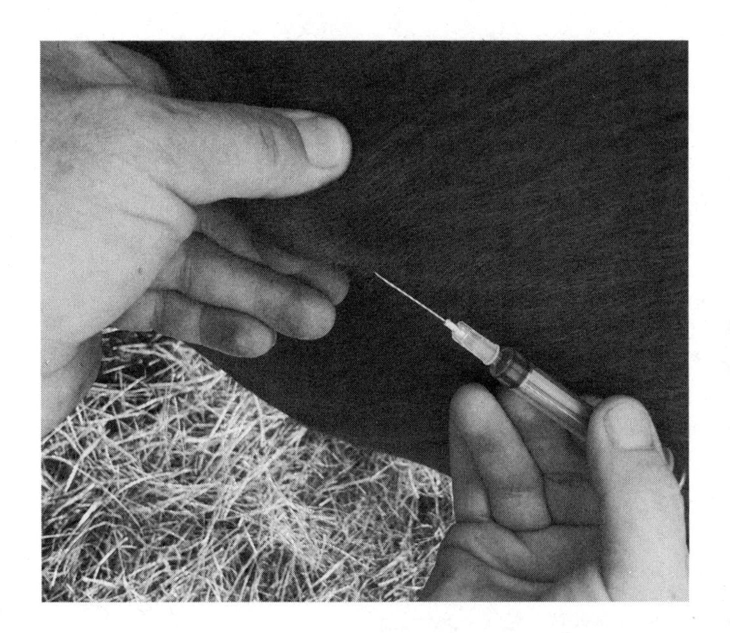

Subcutaneous injection.

Some drugs are given SubQ, which involves pulling up a tent of skin and injecting the drug between the skin and the muscle. This method allows the drug to be absorbed slowly. This is not a hard injection to give, but a steady hand and a quiet cow are necessary to keep from stabbing yourself with the needle. Keep the syringe parallel to the animal and the fold of skin, and depress the plunger smoothly.

Intramuscular injections are the most common. Most antibiotics are given IM, as well as most vaccines. Giving the injection into the muscle tissue allows the drug to be absorbed more quickly than a SubQ injection, due to the muscle having a greater blood supply than the layer under the skin. But the drug is still not absorbed nearly as fast as if it were given IV.

Push the needle firmly into the neck muscle. Injections can be given in the rump, but most producers do not like to use that area. Any time an IM injection is given, it affects the muscle tissue, and when the animal is slaughtered, this might need trimmed away. As the rump produces better cuts of meat than the neck, trimming from neck meat is not as big of a deal.

Needles are designed to be used a single time. When giving shots to a large number of cattle, producers rarely change the needle between each animal. This does save time and money, but the risk of transmitting blood-borne pathogens is increased, as well as causing abscesses from a dirty needle.

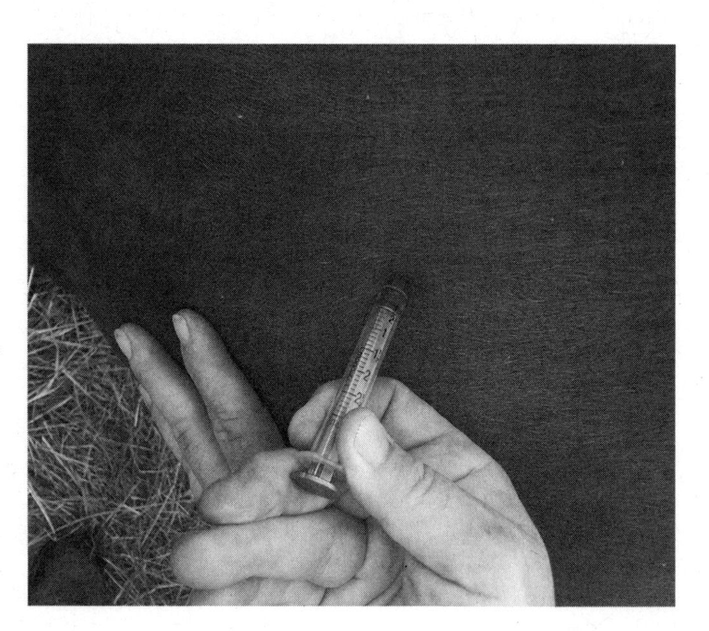

Intramuscular injection.

Needles come in different lengths and sizes. They are given a gauge number, and the smaller the number the larger the diameter. Therefore a 16-gauge needle is much bigger than a 20-gauge.

Antibiotics tend to be rather thick, so most often a larger gauge needle is used, usually a 16. Using a smaller gauge won't let the drug flow through easily, and the animal can get restless. It also takes a lot more pressure to push the plunger down. Some really thick medicines won't flow through a 20-gauge needle at all. On the other hand, using a larger-gauge needle with a less thick liquid means it's possible for some of the medicine to flow back out of the injection hole, resulting in an incomplete dose. Smaller gauge needles are used on calves for obvious reasons.

Needles come in different lengths as well. A short needle, ½ to 1 inch, will work for calves, and a longer one, 1½ inch, will work for adults. Using a short needle on an adult may result in the drug not getting deep enough into the tissue, and a long needle on a calf might do more tissue damage than necessary.

Needles don't actually punch a hole into the skin. They are beveled at the point, and have a cutting edge. This reduces the risk of pushing foreign materials through the skin, and the cut edge closes neatly and cleanly, and heals very quickly.

When you give the injection, give it quickly and smoothly, and don't fish around with the needle too much. That causes unnecessary tissue damage and can result in abscesses.

If you need to give more than 10 mL in any injection, it is best to split the dose up into multiple injection sites. This allows the medication to be absorbed more evenly into the animal's system.

A pistol grip syringe is a great tool for giving multiple injections of the same medication. It can be dosed from 1mL to 5 mL, and when you squeeze the handle, it automatically dispenses the desired dose. It also works well if you have cows that aren't tame or can't be easily handled in a chute. The medication is deposited faster, and there is less chance for tissue damage.

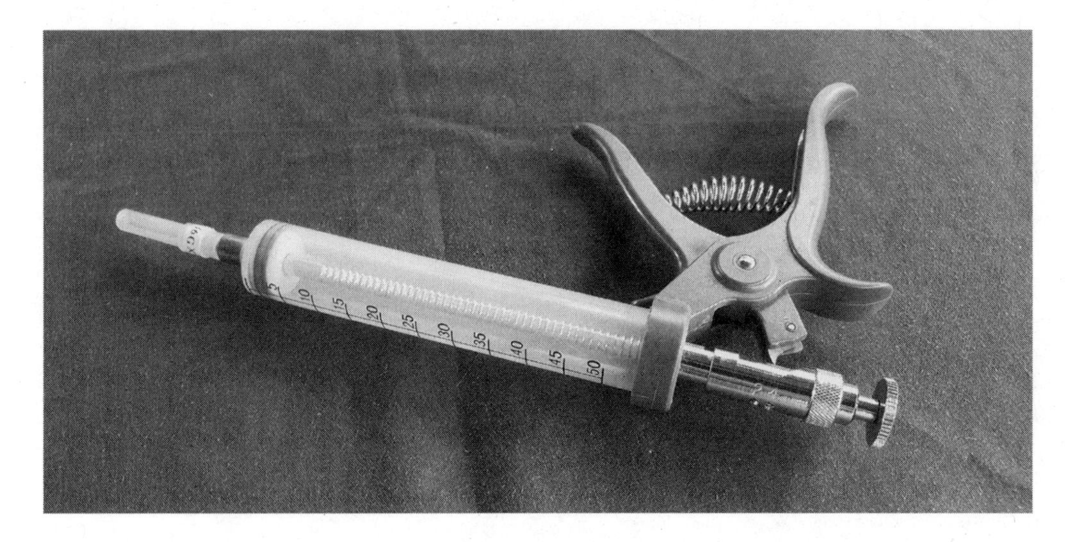

Pistol grip syringe.

4 "Johne's Disease," USDA Animal and Plant Health Inspection Service, June 2020, https://www.aphis.usda.gov/aphis/ourfocus/animalhealth/nvap/NVAP-Reference-Guide/Control-and-Eradication/Johnes-Disease

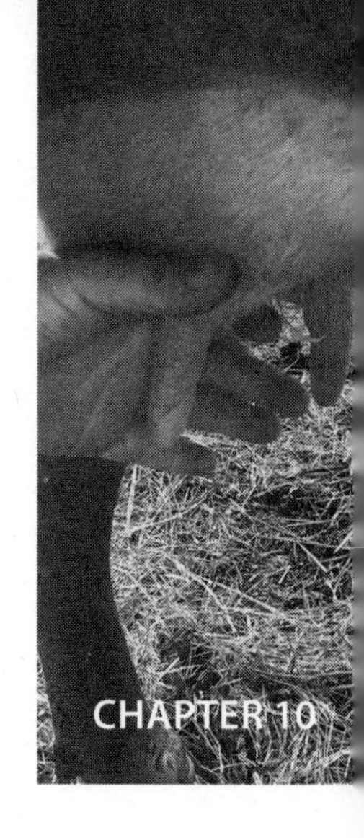

Milk and Milking

Milk has been described as nature's perfect food, and judging by the vast array of cheeses available, it certainly may be. There's no doubt that it is one of our oldest foods, given that archaeological evidence has shown milk and milk product residue in some of the oldest known pottery artifacts.

How the Cow Makes Milk

All cows produce milk, but there is a marked difference between breeds as far as the content of that milk goes. For milk to drink at the table, breed may not matter as much, but if one of your goals is to produce farmstead cheese, yogurt, and other cultured milk products, a breed that produces a richer milk is critical.

As the volume of milk produced goes up, the butterfat content goes down. Jersey cows are known for their butterfat rich milk, Holstein cows for the amazing volume of milk they provide.

Cattle have an udder that is divided by suspensory ligaments into four quarters, each with its own mammary gland system. Each quarter produces and excretes its own milk supply. Udder tissue is made up of a complex system of glands, ducts, and cisterns that hold milk as it is produced until the milk is either nursed by the calf or milked by humans. The udder will become quite distended before it is milked; some high-producing breeds will accumulate 60 to 90 lbs. of milk in the udder before milking.

A complex system of hormones, the chief of which is oxytocin, help trigger creation and let down of milk. If a cow is stressed or startled during the milking process, the surge of adrenaline she experiences will override oxytocin, causing her system of canals and cisterns to clamp down and stop the flow of milk. This doesn't mean you should tiptoe around your cow during milking time, just that it should be as pleasant and stress free as possible.

Milking the Cow

One of the most key components to a successful milking experience is to keep to a strict schedule with your cow as much as humanly possible.

Cattle thrive on routine. If you've ever experienced the severe scolding that comes from being late with an anticipated meal for any livestock, you learn pretty quickly that they tell time better than we do—at least, on some days.

Keeping to a routine is more than just a matter of keeping your animals from being overly dramatic. As the cow learns the routine you've set up, her body and her milk production adapt to what they feel they can expect, and varying milking time or the milking process can make her uncomfortable with an overly full udder or nervous enough to hold back her milk.

In dairies, cattle are milked at minimum twice a day, in some intensive operations three times. They do not raise their calves themselves either; calves are taken away soon after birth and bottle fed. This allows all the cow's milk to be harvested, but it also keeps the calf healthier, since the sheer volume of milk produced by a high-production dairy cow such as a Holstein would more than likely give the calf a severe, and possibly fatal, case of scours.

If the cow is not raising her calf, milking twice a day is essential, and these times need to be spaced as far apart as possible, ideally at least 10 hours apart. If milk is left in the udder, or too much time elapses between milkings, the cow's hormone system takes this as a cue that not as much milk is needed, for whatever reason, and her production will decline.

A cow does not simply "turn on a faucet" and provide a steady supply of milk under any circumstances. Her production will vary depending on how much milk she needs to produce, whether for her calf or for you, and at what point of her lactation cycle she is in. If her udder is not milked down at each milking, it will begin to affect her volume of production, causing her to dry up sooner than you would like.

Also, she does not produce milk forever. At some point, her production will dry up and ultimately cease. She will need to have another calf to start the whole lactation cycle all over again.

One milking option that has become increasingly popular is to share the cow's milk with the calf. This involves leaving the calf and cow together for part of the day, separating them for 10 to 12 hours before the time you want to milk, and then putting them back together again after milking.

The calf can get plenty to eat in the time they are together, and the two will quickly adjust to the routine. Calves raised on their mothers' milk are usually healthier, and this is true even if it's a split schedule. The calf will likely start eating hay and grain sooner and can be weaned sooner.

This approach also reduces the sometimes overwhelming amount of milk that can be produced by a higher-producing breed at peak lactation. And it can give a bit of a breather in your schedule; if you are unable to milk, the calf can remain with the cow instead of being separated; of course, doing this often can affect her production, and she may not produce as much.

The chief thing to keep in mind with a milk cow is that good results will take time, responsibility, and consistency.

Milking Equipment

Basically, the cow is going to have to stand still for the milking process to work. Some cows are great milkers, and you can walk up to them in the pasture and milk them, but most will not allow that, at least not without some training.

At the very least, you will need some sort of simple stanchion, a device that will hold her head, usually while she eats, and will keep her from moving around. She can also be haltered and tied.

Feeding her while she is being milked is a good way to keep her mind off of what you are doing and also serves as a reward for her willing participation in the process.

If she is not willing to let you milk her, especially if she had previously been okay with the process, make sure her udder isn't sore or inflamed. An inflamed udder might be the result of mastitis, improper milking, or injury. The udder will be warm to the touch, and have a hard feeling to it, which is different than the normal, full, ready-to-be-milked feeling.

If her udder is fine, she may just be a reluctant, cranky cow. There are a couple of devices that are designed to keep her from kicking, but they may or may not work, and the cow will need to be restrained to use them.

It is a miserable process to try to milk a cow that isn't willing to be milked. At the least you are more than likely going to lose your pail of milk to a flailing hoof. At worst you may get injured.

Unless the cow is just difficult, most of the time they can be trained to accept milking and even look forward to it. If you have a cow that has never been milked before, or one you are unsure of, spend some time prior to her calving to get her used to the stanchion, or the place she will be milked at. Get her used to being touched and handled, and familiar with people working and moving around her udder and back end.

Raw Milk

The divide between proponents of raw milk and proponents of pasteurization is pretty stark. Raw milk fans claim that milk is sterile coming out of the cow and that pasteurization kills any good probiotics and enzymes in the milk. Advocates for pasteurization claim that pasteurization is the only way to ensure a safe milk supply for the public.

Neither is wrong.

Raw milk was the norm until the late 1800s. Most raw milk was found in the form of yogurt, or clabbered milk. Louis Pasteur developed the pasteurization process in 1864, initially (and perhaps ironically) to increase the keeping quality of wine. At the time, people knew that heat treating certain foods could keep them shelf stable much longer.

In the late 1800s, an increasingly urban population led to the development of what became known as "swill" dairies. These were dairies that were next to alcohol distilleries, and the milk cows were fed the slop left from the brewing process.

The conditions in these dairies were deplorable, the health of the cows nonexistent, and cleanliness unheard of. The milk was watery and unsanitary. In some cases, the infant mortality rate in cities approached 50%, partly due to this poor-quality milk being the only thing available to the poorer classes among the urban population.[5] Enter pasteurization. This process killed bacteria and other harmful organisms in the milk and rendered it safe for human consumption. Infant mortality dropped, and advocates of pasteurization were convinced they had solved the "problem" with raw milk.

By 1910, many cities required milk to be pasteurized, and by 1950 most milk was pasteurized. Gone was the milk delivery man leaving bottles of raw milk from small farms outside the city.

Pasteurization also made an industrial dairy system possible—and inevitable.

Advocates of raw milk argue passionately that milk is basically a sterile perfect food as it comes out of the cow, and the health benefits derived from the enzymes and probiotics found in *properly handled* raw milk *from healthy cows* far outweigh the drawbacks. In either case, whether raw or pasteurized, cleanliness is your best and dearest friend.

Milking Basics

While milk directly out of the cow should be sterile, there are multiple places contamination can occur.

- End of the teat canal
    - The first milk that comes out of the udder will often have been exposed to bacteria. Strip this milk out and do not save it in your milk pail.
- The udder itself
    - As the cow lives her life, mud and manure and other things you don't want in your milk will naturally collect on the udder. Fortunately, cows

out on pasture and not in a dirt lot will have less exposure to contaminants, but still the udder should be thoroughly cleaned before milking.

- Your hands
  - Our own hands are probably one of the biggest vectors for contaminating any food. Be sure to wash your hands whenever handling raw milk, and if you leave the milking area to do something else, wash them before returning to your cow.
- Your facilities
  - Fly control is a must anywhere raw milk will be collected or handled.
  - It's best to have nonporous surfaces whenever possible, but if not, keep the milk area clean, and disinfect with a mild bleach solution.
  - Keep other animals out, and make sure rodent and other pest control measures are in place.

To collect milk, use a stainless steel pail or container. Plastic is porous, and will eventually absorb organic matter into those pores that will be next to impossible to clean out. Glass is also nonporous and a great way to store milk, but has obvious risks out in the barn and around animals.

Clean the cow's udder with warm water, and use a clean cloth every time.

Once the udder is clean, strip a couple of squirts of milk out of each quarter, usually onto the ground—don't allow this to get into your milk pail. Follow up with a teat dip that will kill any remaining bacteria in the teat canal, or on the surface. Strip a couple more squirts out, again onto the ground, and then set to work milking.

It takes a fair amount of hand strength and endurance to milk a cow out by hand. It's also challenging to completely milk out the udder before the cow loses patience: your back and hands give out, and you reconsider moving to the city, especially if you have a heavy-milking breed of cow.

Different people have different aptitudes and abilities to milk. It may be painful for your wrists and hands, but your spouse or kids might be more successful.

There are several "bucket milkers" on the market that are designed to milk a single cow. They come with a milk claw (the part that hooks to the cow) and a stainless steel bucket to catch the milk. The claw is hooked up to an air compressor, causing inflations that squeeze and release, milking out the cow.

There are several advantages to a bucket milker. The milk is contained in the bucket, and not exposed to air or cow hooves. Only the claw is attached to the cow, so she can't kick the bucket over. Used correctly, they milk the cow out quickly and efficiently, making the

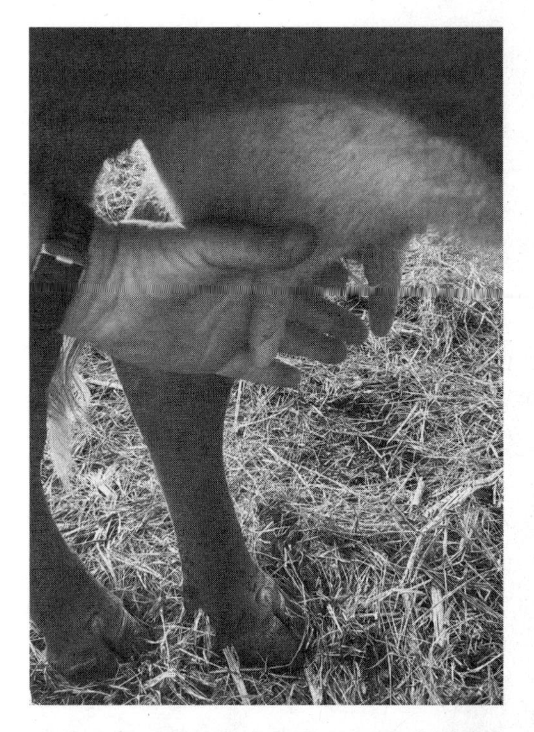

process faster, and it is less likely the cow is going to get bored. It is much easier on your hands.

The downside is, of course, the cost. A bucket milking system can cost a couple of thousand dollars, new. And the equipment must be cleaned and sanitized after each use.

Milk should not be allowed to dry in the equipment. Dried milk film can be very difficult to remove. Rinse the equipment while it's still wet with warm, not hot water. Hot water can "cook" the milk solids and leave them clinging to the system. Milk fat solids are liquid at temperatures above 100°F (37.8°C).

There are several chemicals that are designed for cleaning milk systems.

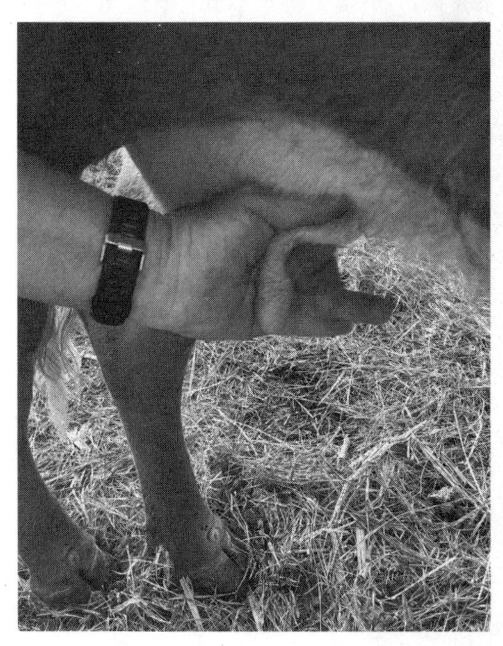

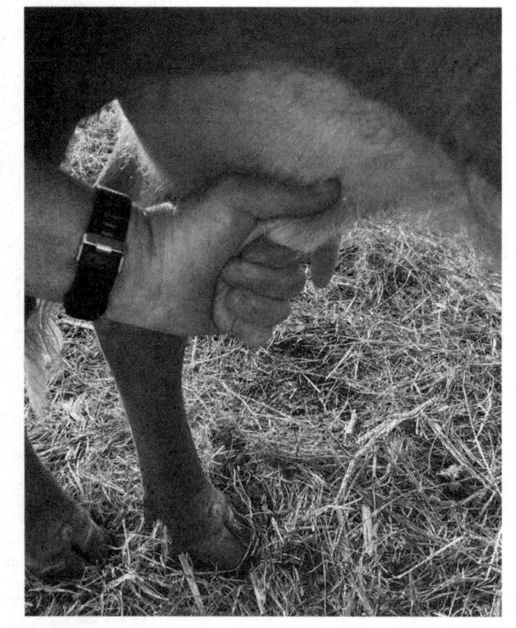

Milking sequence.

Chlorinated alkaline solutions are designed to remove residue of milk from the system. They need to circulate for eight to ten minutes at 165°F (74°C) to be effective. A second rinse, this time with an acid, will remove any hard-water residue, which can give milk something to cling to and promote bacterial growth.

Cleaning and sanitizing a milking system isn't complicated, but the key is to get, and keep, the water at a temperature that will keep the milk fats in a liquid state and enable them to be flushed out of the system. A temperature of 165°F is recommended, and the temperature should not fall below 145°F (63°C). If milk solids collect in the equipment, they are extremely difficult to get out and are prone to bacterial growth, which will then spoil your raw milk.

Handling Raw Milk

After cleanliness, one of the keys to safe raw milk is to get it chilled as soon as possible.

Filter the milk by pouring it through cheesecloth to remove any debris, such as hair, that might have made it into the milk, and get it into storage containers as quickly as possible.

The recommended safe temperature for milk storage is 38°F (3°C). The faster you can get the milk from the cow to that temperature the better off you are. It helps to put the milk into smaller jars or containers; a smaller volume will reach temperature all the way through faster than a larger volume.

If your refrigerator is set to the proper temperature it will work fine for you. Another option is a spare freezer that can be dedicated as just a milk chiller.

A homestead blog I read recommended putting a freezer pack in the milk container while milking to help cool the milk. Personally, this makes me a little nervous, as that pack would have to be kept very, very clean.

Probably the safest and best thing is to get the milk filtered and into pint or quart jars quickly, and then straight into the fridge or freezer.

---

5 Ron Schmid, ND, *The Untold Story of Milk*, 2nd ed., New Trends Publishing, 2009.

Beef

CHAPTER 11

When to Process

THERE'S NO HARD AND FAST RULE for when you should process your beef animal. A variety of factors have to be taken into account, such as the breed of cow, her age, the diet the cow has been on, and so on.

Generally, commercial cattle are slaughtered at about 18 months of age. Much younger and the desired meat-to-bone ratio isn't quite there, much older and the feed costs go up. But for your own farm and your own cow, industry statistics are irrelevant.

Grassfed cattle will take a bit longer to finish, especially if they are totally forage fed. And the length of time will depend on your pasture quality.

Whenever possible, choose a processor close to your farm. The less distance a cow has to be hauled to slaughter, the less stress it will experience and the less shrinkage will occur.

Shrinkage is the weight the animal loses from the time it leaves your farm until the cow is slaughtered. Some will occur naturally as the cow loses belly fill from urinating and defecating, and some will occur as the tissues shrink. The first, excretory shrinkage, will happen regardless of conditions, as the animal does not have access to food or water, but the second, tissue shrinkage, will have more of an impact on the quality of the meat. The longer an animal is in a moving trailer, the more tissue shrinkage will occur. Animals hauled in a trailer for 24 hours will experience an overall weight loss of close to 9% of their starting weight. Cattle lose the most weight in the second and third hours of transit.

If using a small processor, call well in advance of when you think you want to process your beef. Some small processors can be booked months in advance, and you don't want to be ready on your end and have no place to go with your cow.

Small processors usually have only one or two days a week that they will slaughter. This gives them the rest of the work week for cutting up carcasses and making the final product. I've never known one to process on the weekend, so it may be that you need to schedule vacation time to get your animal to the plant.

Generally, they will all have a deadline time that you need to have your animal there by. To keep things moving efficiently on their end, they need to keep things flowing, and they can't stop, unload your cow, and start back up again. Make sure to find out the timing requirements before loading up and leaving home!

Some processors will let you bring your animal in the night before. Ours will let us bring animals in from between 1 and 4 the previous day. The timing ensures the animals have not been without food or water too long.

If you do take your cow in on the day of processing, be sure to take them off feed 12–24 hours prior. This reduces the gut fill and keeps them from urinating and defecating as much, thereby helping to reduce the potential for exposure to contaminants as the animal is processed.

Once you've dropped your cow off, you will give the processor your cut order. The cut order specifies which steaks you want, which roasts, how much ground, etc. If you don't know what to choose, most processors have a standard cut order that you can go by. This usually includes the most common roasts and steaks, and then anything that is left over goes into ground beef. If you're still unsure, the processor is usually happy to answer questions and make suggestions.

So, how much meat can you expect to get? Dress weight is the weight of the carcass after the head and the entrails are removed. This usually averages from 58% to 66% of the live weight. A lot of factors go into this percentage, such as the frame size of the animal, how much muscle and fat it has, and how much gut fill at time of slaughter.

Some of this percentage will include bone, and fat that may be trimmed off the cuts of meat. If you should choose to have the animal made entirely into ground

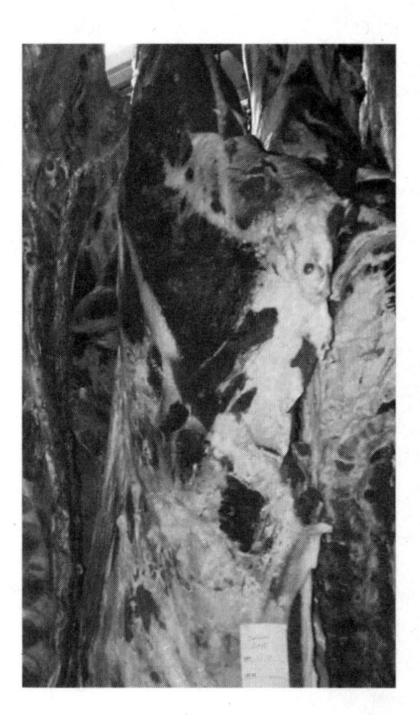

Hanging beef.

beef, expect to have about 35–40% in actual meat. It's hard to find statistics on this because the majority of people don't have their entire cow ground up, but it's been a pretty consistent experience for me over years of slaughtering a variety of species on our farm.

Depending on the processor, there will be a set fee for killing the animal, breaking it down, and disposing of the inedible parts. Some will include their standard cuts in the processing cost, and others will add a fee for doing certain cuts or for grinding some into hamburger. Most usually charge per pound to make specialty products like summer sausage, brats, franks, and anything that has extra labor involved. All processing costs will need to be paid when you pick your meat up.

You can, of course, do your own processing at home. This is admirable, and ambitious, and it's completely out of my scope to advise you on it. If you've hunted and processed your own deer or elk, you are probably better equipped to handle the task than if you haven't had that experience. If you do decide to handle it yourself, ask for help. Seriously, it's a tremendous amount of work, and you need to be efficient. Once that animal is no longer living, the clock is ticking on getting the carcass broken down and chilled as quickly as possible. The longer it goes without being chilled to 38°F (3°C), the more risk of spoilage and food-borne illness.

Freezer Space

An often-quoted statistic is one cubic foot of freezer space for 35–40 lbs. of beef. In my opinion, the meat would have to be so precisely portioned and wrapped to fit that much into that space that I can't see it working well in practice. Meat packages are often oddly shaped. This can be a good thing, since space around the freezer contents will keep them from freezing together and ensure that everything freezes adequately.

I have never taken the measurements on our freezers and how much meat I can stuff into any of them. Usually, I'm in a hurry to get the meat unloaded and stored, and I don't think I've ever had a completely empty freezer that I could start from scratch with.

Some sites that sell freezer beef have recommendations for their customers on freezer size that range from 10 cubic feet for a 100–130 lb. quarter to 4 cubic feet for an 85 lb. quarter. Either of those estimates is way off from 1 cubic foot for 40 lbs. of beef.

An infographic from the University of Minnesota Extension Service shows for a quarter of beef, weighing 142 lbs. (1,300 lb. liveweight) that a 4.5 cubic foot chest freezer or a 5.5 cubic foot upright will be sufficient, and those measurements seem the most reasonable to me.

Chest freezers will hold more because they can be packed more densely. They can also be more of a pain when you are standing on your head trying to get to the bottom, because they can be packed more densely. It's a little easier to organize an upright freezer, but an upright can't be packed as tightly because you want to avoid an avalanche of frozen meat when you open the door.

Beef Cuts

A beef carcass is divided into eight major sections, called primals. The primals are then further broken down into the cuts, or individual roasts or steaks. Different primals had different functions in life, so there can be quite a bit of variability in the tenderness and amount of connective tissue in the resulting meat.

And an animal that lived its life walking around in pasture, as opposed to standing at a feedbunk, will have very different properties. Muscles were meant to work, and as they work they become stronger and are therefore a bit different to chew.

I hesitate to use the words "tender" and "chewy," as the one tends to have a positive connotation and the other a negative. As a society, we've become accustomed to feedlot beef, which is from relatively young animals that haven't moved around much and have been fed a diet intended to produce maximum marbling.

Grassfed beef will be different. It will have a different flavor profile, and as the animal has walked around rather than standing in one place most of its life, its

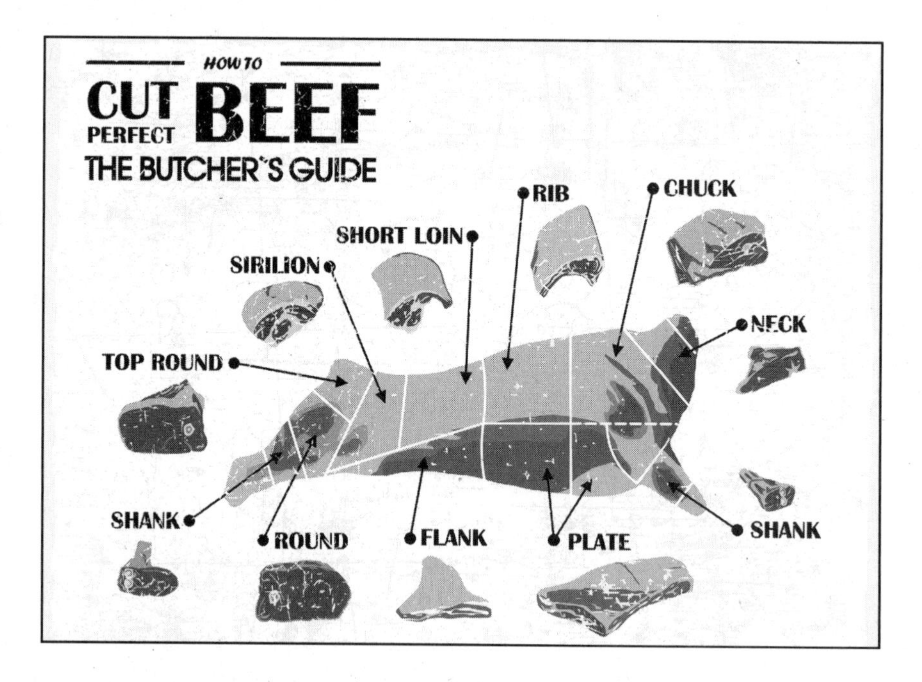

Beef primals guide.

muscle tissue will have developed differently. And, in some instances, it may well take more effort to chew. But, that's why we have teeth, isn't it?

Primals

Chuck

Starting from the front of the carcass the top section, which consists of the neck and the shoulder, is called the chuck. The chuck is a large primal and makes up about 26% of the animal's weight. Because the shoulder is a hard-working group of muscles, the chuck has a great deal of connective tissue. The meat is usually very flavorful, though. Chuck and other cuts with a lot of connective tissue work well with moist cooking methods, such as stewing and braising.

Some chuck cuts include

- Arm roast or chuck roast
- Blade steak
- Stew meat
- Short ribs
- Seven- bone pot roast

Brisket

The brisket is the lower part of the chest of the animal and the foreshanks. Again, as the front legs have done a bit of walking in their lives, the foreshank has a lot of connective tissue. Crosscut foreshanks are one of my favorite cuts of meat; they are flavorful and full of collagen, and, when cooked in an electric pressure cooker, all of that collagen converts to gelatin and makes wonderful soup stock. For some reason, our processor labels this cut as "soup bones" which confused the life out of me initially. The brisket is another cut that is best suited for moist heat cooking, such as simmering or braising.

Some brisket cuts include

- Shank cross cuts
- Flat cut brisket

Rib

The rib primal, is the section immediately behind the chuck, makes up about 10% of the carcass weight. Two of the best-known cuts of meat from the rib primal are the rib roast (prime rib) and the ribeye steak. This center muscle provides structural support, not mobility, and is therefore very tender and may be more marbled than the rest of the carcass.

Some rib cuts include

- Rib roast
- Rib steak
- Ribeye steak
- Ribeye roast

Short Plate and Flank

Located directly beneath the ribs, the short plate and flank are meaty but full of connective tissue. Flank steak is a paddle-shaped cut of meat with a long grain that works wonderfully for marinating and searing. Often the short plate is used for ground beef.

Some plate and flank cuts

- Skirt steak
- Flank steak
- Hanger steak

Short Loin

The short loin resides just behind the rib section and, while making up only 8% of the carcass weight, is home to many of the most tender, and expensive, cuts. It is also a primal where the cuts are all somewhat interrelated. The tenderloin is the most tender cut and can be taken out whole or cut into tenderloin steaks, also known as filet mignon. The popular T-bone and porterhouse steaks also come from this area, so if you want a tenderloin, you will not be able to have those steaks. New York strip steaks also come from this primal and are taken from the loin eye muscle running along the top of the back. Porterhouse and T-bone steaks both have a portion of the New York Strip on one side and the tenderloin on the other; the T-bone will come from the front of the loin area, the Porterhouse from the rear, where it will have a larger portion of the tenderloin.

Loin cuts include

- Porterhouse steak
- T-bone steak
- Tenderloin roast
- Tenderloin steak

Sirloin

The sirloin is located behind the short loin and before the rump. Sirloin cuts are not as tender as those from the short loin, but they are meaty flavorful cuts. There are several names for the sirloin steaks and roasts, but all do best with dry heat cooking methods like broiling, grilling, or roasting.

Sirloin cuts include

- Sirloin steak
- Tri-tip roast
- Tri-tip steak

Round

The round is a very large primal, approximately 27 % of the carcass weight. Round cuts include minute steak (which is usually tenderized and is often used for chicken fried steak), round roasts, and hindshanks. Because the round contains less fat content than other primals, it will require low and slow cooking, or marinating prior to cooking.

Round cuts include

- Round steak
- Round tip roast
- Bottom round roast

Cattle and the Environment

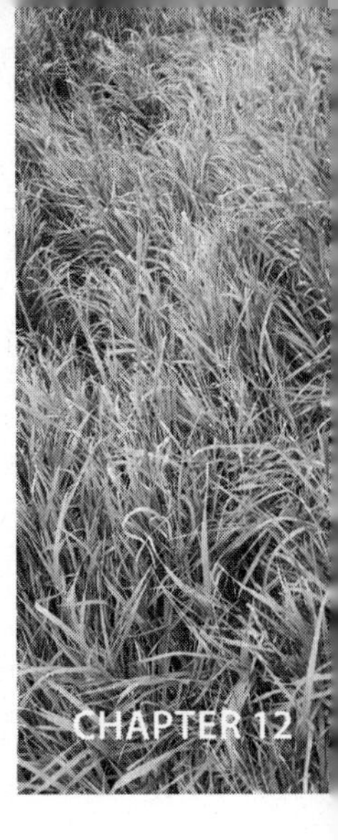

GUESS WHAT?

Cow farts aren't really ruining the world. There are a whole lot of other things that are, but at least as far as our cows are concerned, they play a rather small part. And besides, they don't fart methane, they belch it.

But I digress.

In 2006, the Food and Agriculture Organization (FAO) released a mammoth 400-page report, titled *Livestock's Long Shadow* (LLS), on the perceived impact of livestock on climate-change issues globally. In that report, livestock were blamed for 18% of greenhouse gas emissions. The whole world pretty much lost its mind over the report, and cattle became the climate-change whipping boy.

Subsequent research and criticism of the original report revealed that there were some inconsistencies in the data used to come up with the 18% emissions estimate. For one, in calculating the transportation numbers, only tailpipe emissions were used, compared to a complete life cycle analysis for livestock.

In 2015, Frank Mitloehner, a professor and air quality specialist at the University of California-Davis published a criticism of the data used in LLS, finding the percentage of greenhouse gas emissions directly contributable to livestock closer to 4.2%, a huge difference. Even one of the authors of *Livestock's Long Shadow* admitted that Mitloehner had a legitimate criticism of their data and findings.

Unfortunately, the popular media, never inclined to miss a good sensation, seized on the original numbers, and they have now been used so much that they seem to have taken root and have been tough to dislodge. Campaigns such as "Meatless Monday" continue to still tout the statistic as if it were indisputable fact.

Arguments to completely do away with livestock and feed people on the grains used to feed animals also have root in some pretty powerful misconceptions and have become loaded emotional issues for proponents. When emotion holds sway, logic has a hard time getting its foot in the door.

There is little doubt that the modern livestock industry does contribute to greenhouse gas emissions, but as with most other industries, the bulk comes from transportation factors, not the animals themselves.

Another commonly made mistake is to lump all livestock into the same bucket, but in reality there are a huge variety of production systems, goals, and methods, from small farms with a half dozen animals to huge confinement operations, and everything in between.

Back in the millennia before domestication took place, much of the world, and especially the Great Plains of the United States, were covered with grass. This grass evolved along with species that could use the grass—having developed the specialized digestive capacity to make use of what would otherwise be indigestible material. Huge herds of bison and other ruminants grazed on these prairies, nipping off grass to feed themselves and depositing their manure to feed the grass.

Grass does not do well without grazers. It becomes overgrown, stemmy, and eventually can choke itself out. Grazing animals take the tops of the grass and move along, stimulating the plants to put on new growth and store photosynthetic energy in their roots, to draw from the next time they get grazed.

Grazing also led to the development of rich, fertile soil, which early settlers were all too keen to capitalize on for planting crops, and thus a vicious cycle was born.

Plowing up grassland removes the hold provided by the elaborate root systems of the grass and opens the soil to erosion. The bare soil left behind lets carbon escape into the atmosphere, contributing to greenhouse gasses, and a whole host of other detrimental environmental events also begin to occur.

Fortunately, a "new" system of raising livestock has been gaining ground. I put "new" in quotes, because the methods are literally as old as grass itself. Regenerative grazing, holistic grazing, management-intensive grazing, and rotational grazing are all labels that basically describe the same thing: using grass and grazers to improve the soil, and to reduce (!) greenhouse gas emissions through the use of livestock and livestock farming.

One of the most notable advocates of regenerative grazing is Alan Savory, whose work in reclaiming degraded land has created quite a stir in the livestock community. Although Savory is not without his critics, the proof is in the land itself and in the quiet groundswell of cattle producers using rotational grazing and having tremendous success with the methods.

Grassfed Beef

Grassfed beef is experiencing a renaissance as well. At one time, the only beef available was grassfed, and it was finished, processed, and sold locally. Enter the mid-20th century, and four corporate conglomerates dominated the landscape, buying 80% of the cattle on the market.

But more recently, grassfed beef accounted for sales of $272 million in 2016, up from $17 million in 2012.[6]

Of the total percentage of grassfed beef sales, 19% is sold directly from the farmer to the consumer, the other 81% goes into branded programs. Branded programs are companies that purchase beef or beef animals and then market them under their own brand.

While the grassfed beef market is gaining traction, there are a few challenges.

Because the beef is not fed subsidized grain for the final part of its life, and production costs are borne entirely by the farmer, grassfed beef often costs more to purchase.

Feeding cattle on grass through harvest also takes a bit longer than conventional grain-fed beef, and as a result, it can be harder to have a consistent supply to market. And because of the variety of farms and production systems, grassfed beef is not always consistent from one farm to another.

With minor exceptions, all beef cattle start life on pasture. Calves are born and graze with their mothers until they are weaned. From that point, they either continue on pasture as "background" calves or go directly into the feedlot system. Background calves spend a few months more on pasture before going into the feedlot system.

Terms:

Pasture raised: An animal that was raised on pasture until moving onto the feedlot.

Grassfed: Ate grass at some point in its life; may or may not have gone into the feedlot to finish.

Grass finished: An animal that was raised entirely on pasture, and processed directly from pasture. Interestingly enough, there have been a few "grass feedlots" developed lately, where the calf is confined, and fed hay. Not the same as a conventional feedlot but still very different than being out on pasture.

Conventional: The traditional stocker cattle system, from pasture to feedlot and processed within 18–24 months.

There are several organizations that label grassfed beef. One of the oldest and most respected is the American Grassfed Association, which requires that in order to carry the AGA label, the animal must have been fed on grass its *entire* life and been raised on pasture, not confinement.

Grazing Systems

Continuous

In a continuous grazing system, cattle are allowed to graze the entire pasture area as they choose.

The plus to this system is that there is very little labor and very little facility and equipment necessary. There is no requirement for movable fencing, extra water tanks, or any of the other things needed to create a rotational grazing system.

The downside of continuous grazing systems is that ultimately, the cows will overgraze some areas with more preferable forages, while leaving others totally ungrazed. Just because there is a tall stand of grass out there doesn't mean the cow will choose to eat that. Remember as the forage gets taller, the amount of stem increases, the level of nutrition reduces, and the cow will try to graze anything else but those stems.

On a new, or new to you, farm, it may be necessary initially to continuous graze. Unless you have a completely bare property with no previous infrastructure, where you have the option of starting from square one, it will take time to figure out what your plan should be. It will take some time to switch everything over a rotational grazing system.

Rotational Grazing

A rotational grazing system by any other name still performs the same function.

The intention is to give each section of pasture some time to rest and recover after grazing. The recovery time can be a few days or a few weeks, and may or may not be enough to let the grazed portion of the grass fully recover. However, with rest the plant will be able to recover somewhat. How much depends on the season, rainfall, and a variety of other factors that affect plant growth.

Pastures in a rotational grazing system may be permanently fenced or may use temporary fencing.

Management-Intensive Grazing

Management-intensive grazing, or MiG, as its proponents like to call it, is the most intensive of the grazing systems. It is also called high-density grazing, or mob grazing. Whatever name you call the system, it involves temporary fences that are moved daily, or in the case of some systems, every few hours. It also generally involves a larger group of cows.

The goal of MiG grazing is to keep the herd bunched together, moving rapidly over a section of ground. The theory is that when cattle are bunched together, they eat a little more competitively and are motivated to eat anything green before the other cows do.

Their manure is therefore more evenly spread out, and the pasture plants are grazed more uniformly.

As the name implies, the labor and management are more intensive with this system. It takes an experienced eye to be able to monitor the amount of forage grazed and adjust the next paddock up or down in size, depending on what is learned from the previous ones.

The advantages are several: even grazing of pasture; distribution of manure; ample time between grazings, allowing plant recovery; and higher nutrition for the cows, since they have constant access to fresh pasture.

The disadvantages include the time required to move fence regularly and set up water in each paddock. It may not be practical for those with an off-farm job. And it's also possible, depending on the grazing season and the rate at which pasture is growing, to have grass growing faster than the cows can graze it, at least before it becomes stemmy and goes to seed.

With any system, there are a lot of variables. The amount of rainfall may change from year to year, resulting in different growth rates at the same time of year. What worked last year may not work this year. Grazing management requires constant tweaking and time to observe and make management decisions. In fact, without time to look and think and plan, an intensive grazing system may do more harm than good.

Some sort of pasture rotation is necessary to prevent overgrazing and maximize the nutrition your cows can receive from the pasture. And, as drought becomes more and more prevalent, being able to rest pastures is critical to their long-term health. Don't expect to become an expert overnight. Observe, and be willing to change and tweak strategies to work with whatever Mother Nature throws at us from year to year.

Making It Work for One Cow

The majority of the informational resources on rotational grazing involve working with large herds, mostly of commercial cows, and making use of quite large sections of land where it is possible to divide the pasture into multiple paddocks. For a larger herd, it makes sense to spend the money involved in setting up the infrastructure and water supply systems to support it. It can be part of the strategy and plan to sell cows when pasture resources are scarce and/or to purchase extra calves or stocker cattle when grass is abundant.

For those of us with just a handful of cows, a single cow that we milk, or a conservation breeding herd, it will never be quite that simple. The principles of grazing management can translate for a smaller herd just as effectively but with a few minor tweaks.

A key concept is to get a good feel for how fast your pasture is recovering. If the weather is dry, or if it is later in the grazing season, when growth has naturally slowed, you may have to adjust your strategy. If it is not recovering as fast as conditions are requiring rotation, have a sacrifice area set up where you can feed hay when necessary and give the pasture time to recover.

Take into account what your cow's nutritional needs are. If she's in peak lactation or just calved and her needs are high, graze her then, and feed hay when she's not on such a high nutritional plane.

Bear in mind that not only are we trying to make the best use of our grass for the cow's benefit, but we are also trying to make that grass as healthy as possible so it can do its work of reducing erosion, sequestering carbon, enriching the soil, and being a truly renewable resource.

How Grass Grows

Grass is really pretty cool stuff. It takes sunlight and, by the magic of photosynthesis, turns what could otherwise be wasted energy into forage that animals can utilize. We all learned about photosynthesis in elementary school science. That may have been a while ago, so, just as a refresher:

Sunlight hits the grass. Grasses and other plants have chlorophyll, which captures that sunlight, takes carbon dioxide (CO_2) and water, and turns them into carbohydrates and oxygen. Chlorophyll is also what gives plants their green color. The system is in reality much, much more complicated than that, but the basic truth is that grass takes sunlight and turns it into carbohydrates. Sunlight falling on bare ground is wasted because there is nothing green to capture it and turn it into usable energy.

If the energy created by photosynthesis is not needed for the plant to grow, it will store the excess carbohydrates in its roots. This reserve storage of energy is vitally important for the plant to survive. Without it, once the top of the grass is grazed off, the plant has less leaf surface with which to photosynthesize. It needs those reserves to help regrow the grass leaf so that photosynthesis can take over again.

If grass is grazed too short, it must use more of its root reserve to regrow the leaves. If a portion of the grass leaf is left after grazing, it can use photosynthesis, and not have to take as much from its root reserve. And the grass can't store new root reserves until the leaves regrow.

The most vigorous regrowth occurs when less than 50% of the top is taken off, and the more leaves left on the plant, the more it is able to photosynthesize.

Younger leaves are more efficient at photosynthesis as well. As the plant matures and enters the reproductive phase, characterized by putting on a seedhead, it is characterized by more stem and less leaf and is therefore less efficient at photosynthesis.

Types of Grasses

There are two types of grasses: warm season and cool season. Each is characterized by the season at which it is most active.

Cool-season grasses, such as brome, are more active when the temperature is around 65–75°F (18–24°C). Cool-season grasses are the first to start growing in the spring but become dormant in warmer weather. They will also, unless they have been cut or grazed, go to seed before the weather gets too hot. Cool-season grasses will often experience a regrowth in the fall, once the summer heat has passed, given that there is sufficient rainfall.

Warm-season grasses, such as fescue and big bluestem, have the opposite growth pattern. They grow best when temperatures are in the 90–95°F range (32–35°C). In fact, they will not really grow at all until the soil temperature reaches around 60°F (15°C). And, when the weather begins to cool off, they will become dormant.

An ideal pasture would have a mix of both grasses, so that when one is beginning to slow its growth, the other will be coming on.

Grazing Behavior

Unlike goats, which have a small, nimble muzzle and lips, cattle have a large, rather fixed mouth and lips. While a goat can nibble the choicest leaves, the cow is limited to what she can scoop into her mouth with her tongue.

Cattle have no upper front teeth, just a hard palate. This limits how close they can normally graze plants, making them much kinder to a pasture than, say, a horse.

With their large rumen, cattle will graze for a period of time, until that rumen is full, and then lie down to rest and ruminate. If the forage they are grazing is of good quality, the rumen will be able to provide the cow, and the bacteria in the rumen, with a lot of high-quality energy and protein. Should the forage be of lower quality, with more stem or less nutritious grass, the bacteria and cow will not have taken in enough to maintain their needs.

If pastures are of sufficient height, the cow will move along, grazing the tops of the forage, and she can take in more per bite. In shorter pastures, the cow has to work a little harder with each bite, and as we saw in Chapter 9, in the section on parasites, the taller grass will keep her from grazing down to the height at which parasite larvae can migrate.

As the cow moves through the pasture, she inevitably steps on plants, or the remainders of plants. Her cloven hoof flexes and twists, cutting plant material and grinding it into the ground.

Sounds awful, right? It isn't!

Healthy grass depends on healthy soil, which depends on organic matter decomposing to provide nutrients. In order for the bacteria that decompose plant material to be able to do so, the plant material must be in contact with the ground. As the cow walks through the pasture, her feet press that plant material into the ground, where bacteria can break it down, and it can be used to increase the nutrient level of the soil, thereby helping fuel the next generation of grass plants.

It's the same cycle that built the prairies over millennia. The bovine grazes, tramples, defecates, and then moves on, no matter whether it was a bison before the 19th century or a domestic cow.

The problem comes around when the cow tramples the same area over and over again. As that happens, the amount of good grazing material that is ground into the soil increases past the point of recovery. This is another reason why resting pastures between grazings is so vital to healthy pastures. It prevents healthier grass from being damaged and allows the soil microbes to do their work.

As large herds, pre-domestication, moved through the prairie, they moved in tight bunches, keeping close together to avoid predators. As they moved through, they kept moving and did not re-graze where they had defecated. This allowed the manure to break down and the cycle to be completed before the forage was grazed again. Moving on rather than grazing in one place helped keep parasite loads low as well.

By the same token, as cows move through pasture they leave manure behind. And as with pre-domestic herds, the manure provides a nice, moist environment for the bacteria to do their thing, and bacteria shed from the rumen enhance the bacteria populations in the soil. Bacteria and their activity are fundamental to the cycle of life. Without them to break down organic material and turn it into nutrients for the grass, the entire life cycle on our planet would break down dramatically.

Implementing a Grazing Plan

Figuring out what to do starts with a good look at what you have. Take some time to take a good honest look at your pastures. If possible, spend some time during a range of seasons to see how things grow. What looks green and lush during April and May may not look so great when August rolls around.

Making a plan that includes worst-case scenarios, at least as far as rainfall and weather are concerned, will keep you from spending more than you planned on hay or having to part with your cows.

Good Pastures

Good pastures will be lush. Grass will be thick, and very few bare spots will be seen. You should see a variety of plant species. In a managed hay meadow you should definitely have more grass, as a rule, but in a pasture that will be grazed a variety of species help keep diversity thriving, and many plants thought of as weeds can actually be beneficial and nutritious.

Good pasture systems will also build in a sacrifice area. A sacrifice area is exactly that, an area separated from the rest of the pasture where livestock can be put when conditions are not optimal for grazing, such as the rainy season, winter, or drought. Because they will be concentrated in one spot in less-optimum weather or rainfall conditions, they will damage the plants and possibly kill them, depending on type. But better a small area heavily damaged than less damage spread throughout your entire pasture.

How will your cattle get water? A grazing plan should not depend on animals drinking from ponds or creeks, not unless there is some effort to mitigate the damage they can do to stream banks or pond shores.

Poor Pastures

By contrast, poor pastures are prone to weeds like ragweed, thistle, and other noxious plants. Bare spots might be common. If cattle have been on this pasture previously, it might be overgrazed in some places and underutilized in

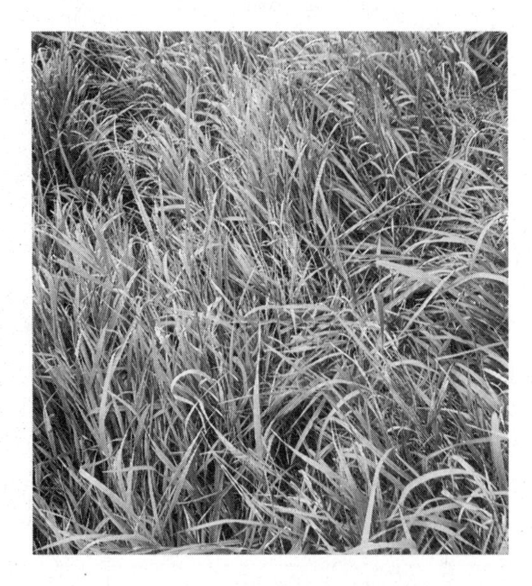

A good stand of Brome grass.

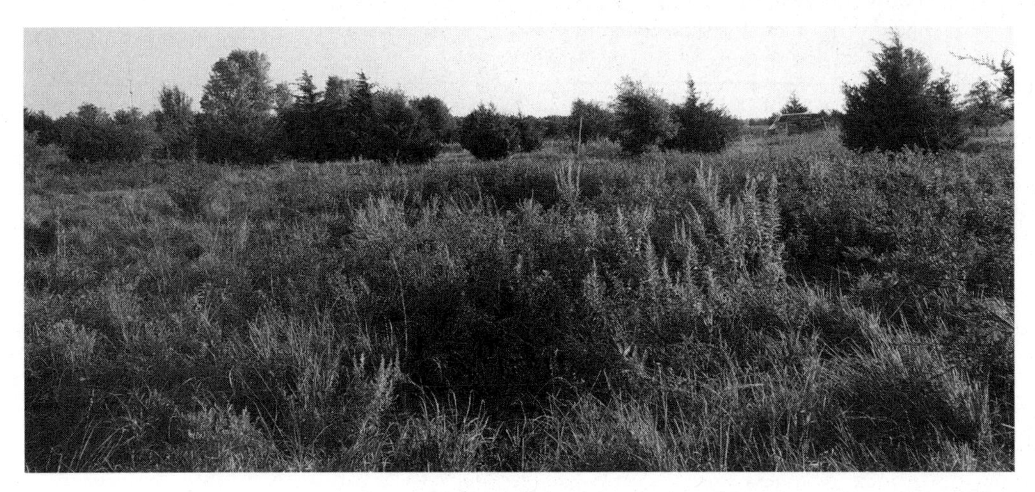

Pasture that has been undergrazed.

others. Cattle love the tender goodness of young grass shoots and will graze back over areas before they have adequate time to recover. This starts the downward spiral of plants not being able to store and conserve the resources they need for optimum regrowth. It also leaves places with taller, less palatable grass that they will ignore in favor of the tender little nibbles. Once grass reaches a certain level of stemminess and lignin content, cattle will be reluctant to touch it.

Poisonous Weeds Chart

Poke Weed	Roots and berries most toxic. Can cause abortion in cows.
Johnson Grass	Poisoning due to increased accumulation of nitrates.
Poison Hemlock	Dangerous but rarely eaten. Leaves and unripe fruit are poisonous.
Nightshade	Leaves and unripe fruit are highly poisonous.
St. Johns Wort	Causes photosensitization, inflammation of pink skin, which may peel and slough.
Pigweed (several species)	All parts of plant are dangerous. Results in cardiac arrest 5–10 days after eating.
Jimsonweed	All parts toxic, especially seeds. As little as .06% of body weight can be fatal to cattle.
Cocklebur	Seeds and young seedlings highly poisonous. Death is rapid, within 12–24 hours.
Black Locust	Bark, roots, seeds, and wilted leaves are toxic.

If a water source is present in the pasture, and cattle have had unrestricted access to it, it might be degraded.

Never fear, all these problems can be improved with careful management. A badly abused pasture may take quite some time to recover, but a good grazing plan can begin to help turn things around almost immediately.

Evaluating Pastures

Plants

Step one is to figure out what plant species you are working with. Your local extension office will often have guides that can help you identify species, both weeds and desirable plants.

In the modern internet age, there is no shortage of websites and apps that can help identify plants. One I have found particularly useful is the Seek app, by iNaturalist. It has so far proved the most reliable and user friendly of all the ones I've tried. (I haven't tried many—once I found Seek I became a loyalist.) I also appreciate that it identifies insects, reptiles, and amphibians as well. Having a diverse healthy pasture means there is a home for these critters as well, so it's great to see who we share the farm with. Seek also stores your observations in the app, so you can refresh yourself on what's what and keep a running checklist of the species you've identified.

Taking stock of what is actually growing in your pastures can help inform your

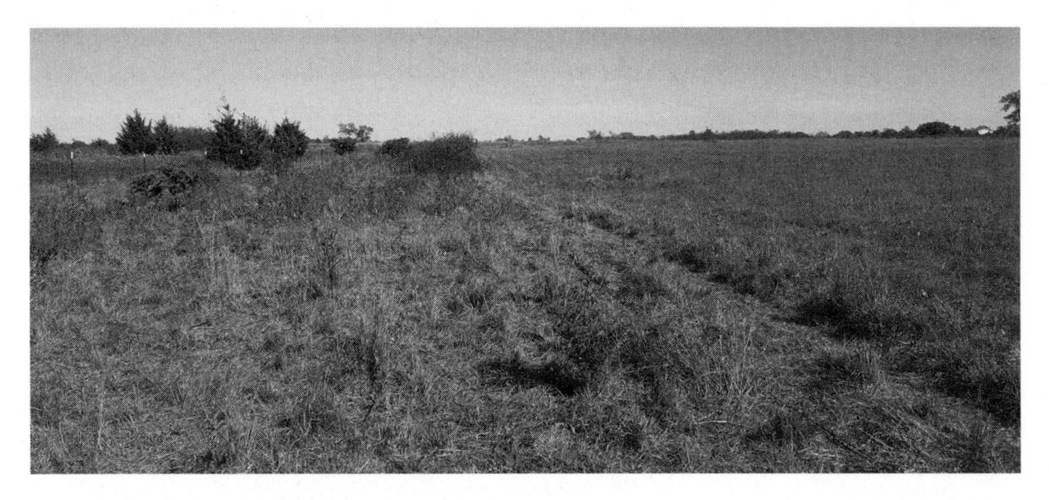

Contrast between poorly managed pasture and rotationally grazed.

first steps. If you find a variety of plants that are considered toxic, the first thing to do is remove those. Weeds do not tolerate being mowed repeatedly, so the first step might be to mow or physically remove them. Weeds can be tenacious, though. Some have complex root systems that can send out shoots and pop up elsewhere nearby. Keeping up with mowing and weed control will weaken them each time, though, and eventually you can get ahead of them. Remember that weeds can be crowded out by healthy grass too, so keeping the pasture properly grazed or mowed can eventually reduce them to a bad memory.

Sensitive Areas

No, I'm not necessarily talking about hurting their feelings. But streams and ponds are areas that will need careful management. Allowing cattle unrestricted access to streams will degrade banks, cause erosion, dirty the water, and generally undo any environmental good you are trying to do. Ponds and streams can be used to water cattle, but it requires attention. Cattle can be fenced away from ponds and allowed access to water only at certain points; the same with streams.

Wetlands and marshy areas are also places that should be taken into consideration when evaluating how to implement your plan.

Fences

A good, substantial perimeter fence is a must. It doesn't have to be strong enough to hold an elephant, but it should be well maintained, and wires should be tight and anchored to fenceposts. It shouldn't sag, or have gaps that a calf could squeeze through. Barbwire is a common cattle fence and works well when it's tight. In the case of some older barbwire fences that have not been maintained, it's not unusual for the lower wires to have gotten loose from the posts and be lying on the ground covered by grass. Cattle are pretty good about not getting tangled in wire, but the potential still exists for animals to get injured by loose wire.

Smooth wire looks great, but cattle are not known for respecting it unless it is electrified. And electric fence is not a great choice for a perimeter fence. The potential is always there for it to get grounded out, and the chance that cows will escape is too much of a risk.

The perimeter fence will be the boundary for all the subdivisions you will create when you develop your grazing plan, so it definitely needs to be in good repair.

Water

Water, or access to it, is possibly the most important consideration when laying out your grazing plan. How will you get water to your livestock when they are grazing at the far end of your system? Make sure you plan a system that won't have you frustrated halfway through the grazing season.

Hopefully, you will not be grazing much during the colder months of the year, and allowing your pastures to rest. Trying to get water to livestock at the far end of a pasture during freezing weather is a challenge I'm not brave enough to tackle. We bring our cattle in to a central lot and sacrifice area to feed them hay, and it has a central tank that is served by a hydrant. It also has power at the hydrant for a tank heater.

Fortunately, there are a variety of solar options for tank heaters and aerators that will keep ponds and tanks from icing up in all but the most extreme cold, if having power at your water source isn't an option.

Soil Quality

A soil sample can give you some idea whether you need to consider adding fertilizer. If pastures are heavily degraded, or soil quality is poor, an application of fertilizer can help you get a jump start on your grazing program. Fertilizers are relatively inexpensive for the material itself. Having it professionally applied may or may not be an additional option for you, depending on the geography of your pasture. Your local extension service can point you in the direction of a soil test and help you to figure out a plan. Timing is also critical in the application of fertilizers. The last thing you want to do is apply fertilizer only to watch it run into the stream or pond in a heavy spring thunderstorm.

Creating a Sacrifice Area

Your next step will be to choose a dedicated sacrifice area. This area will spare your pastures in times when you can't, or shouldn't, graze.

Unless you live in that rare unicorn of a climate where you have grass growing year-round, there will be times when you can't graze. In the vast majority of cases, you will also need to feed hay in the winter.

Drought is also an ever-increasing possibility in our modern climate, where the trend is unfortunately slanting toward instability. Having an area that allows you to spare your pastures until the rains (hopefully) come again will keep them from being overgrazed and damaged.

Rainy seasons are also a time the sacrifice area can be invaluable. Mud compacts easily under cow hooves, damaging the plants and their roots, and doing more damage than just about any other weather condition.

Depending on your type of forage, it will be difficult for you to graze through the winter. Plant growth naturally slows down in the winter, and grazing during the winter can reduce forage growth later, as the plants will have lost their reserves needed to fuel growth in the spring. And it can't be said too often: overgrazing stresses plants.

Deciding Paddock Size

Determining the size of the subdivisions in your pasture is easier if you are starting with a bare acreage, but that isn't always an option. Also, the optimal paddock size will more than likely vary from year to year, depending on the weather and the amount or lack of rainfall.

Dividing a pasture into paddocks will increase the forage yield of the land dramatically—up to a point. The best increases in forage yield will come with the initial subdivisions. You will likely see a dramatic increase in the forage output. But after a certain point the grass can only grow so much, and continuing to further subdivide may not provide enough return to justify the labor.

This is the time to really evaluate and consider your goals. If you are planning a small-scale dairy, your management will need to be a little more intensive than if you are just planning to raise a few animals for beef.

Lactating dairy cows have one of the highest nutritional needs of any class of livestock. In some intensive grazing systems, dairy cows are moved a couple of times a day to keep them on the best forage available.

The number of paddocks available to you will also depend on the rest interval your pasture needs. When planning your system, base your math around the longest regrowth period, not the shortest. This should be late summer for most of us, but climate variability can trigger this earlier in the season than we might expect. For example, in Kansas, the native prairie grass wakes up in late April and early May and grows rapidly (depending on available moisture) and may be able to recover in as short a time as two weeks. It will continue its growth through the hot part of the summer, although as July and August get drier, not as fast. The length of rest needed may increase to 21–30 days. In times of drought, it might take 45–60 days for the pasture to recover enough to tolerate grazing.

Unfortunately, there is no tried-and-true formula other than good observation and being willing and able to react when things aren't going as planned.

Find an old yardstick. Walk out into the pasture on a regular basis, and measure how much regrowth has occurred. Note it on a calendar, and check it again in a week. Most grazing experts recommend never grazing shorter than 4 inches and, in the case of native prairie, closer to 6 inches.

If you begin to see bare patches in your pasture, or uneven forage height, it's time to give the pasture a much longer rest time, perhaps even a season, so that the plants can rebuild their reserves.

If you underestimate the regrowth time, pastures will not have recovered sufficiently. If you overestimate, pastures will overgrow and the grass will become less palatable, but the plants will at least be healthy.

Decide how many days you will let the cows graze each paddock. Be honest with yourself. Do not construct small paddocks planning to move cows daily if you know that's just not going to work with your schedule. If you have an off-farm job, and your luck is like mine, having a farm task you absolutely need to do after work is a signal to the universe to unleash a crisis at work.

Some rotation is better than none. Three days on a paddock seems to be the maximum to prevent overgrazing. But, if you know the only time you will be able to move cows is on the weekends, plan for a 7-day grazing rotation. No, it's not ideal, but we all do the best we can. Don't let the perfect become the enemy of the good.

If you leave your cows on one paddock for 10–14 days, however, you will find half the grass overgrazed, and half undergrazed. The overgrazed will have poor regrowth.

The formula:

Number of paddocks = (days rested / days grazed) +1

The extra day accounts for always having an empty paddock to move to.

So, for example, if you know you will be able to move the cows only every third day, and the maximum period for regrowth during late summer is 42 days, this is the formula

42 / 3 = 14 + 1 = 15 paddocks.

OK, great. Now, how big do those paddocks need to be?

This is where it gets a little more complicated, and a variety of regional factors come into play. You will need to know how much mass per acre your pasture will produce and how much forage your herd requires on a daily basis. Fortunately, there are already studies done to determine this on a variety of forages.

Livestock will consume 2.5% of their body weight daily, which is the general rule of thumb in most nutritional charts. That is the number I used in the following examples, but as you begin planning your pasture paddock sizes, experiment with adding .5% or 1% to your calculations. This can give you a buffer to avoid overgrazing as you start out. Once you get a feel for your pasture and what works for you, you will develop your own rules of thumb. Many factors will affect how well any plan works, so these examples are just examples—a place to begin. Grazing is both science and art.

So, if you have cows that average 1,350 lbs. then 2.5% = 34 lbs. of forage per day. If your forage produces 1,250 lbs. of DM per acre, and you have 50 head of cattle, and you plan for a two-day grazing stay, then

34 lbs. × 50 head = 1,700 lbs. forage for the group per day.

For two days, 1,700 × 2 = 3,400 lbs. total.

If your forage produces 1250 lbs. per acre, 3,400 / 1,250 = 2.72 acres needed for each paddock.

So, if you need 15 paddocks to allow for your 42-day rest interval, and each paddock needs to be 2.72 acres, then 15 × 2.72 = 40.8 acres total is how much pasture you need to be able to pull it off.

There are lots of ways to tweak the math.

If 50 cows are a lot, try 25.

a 1,350-lb. cow is pretty big—go for a smaller breed.

An 800-lb. cows at 2.5% of their body weight will only eat 20 lbs. of forage instead of 34. So right there, 25 × 20 lbs. = 500 lbs. forage. At the same forage productivity and length of time in paddock, 1,000 lbs. of forage is needed. So, 1,000 / 1,250 per acre = 0.8 acre paddocks. And 15 paddocks is 12 acres, at this rate. Of course, this math can be somewhat misleading; allowance must be made for lanes; sacrifice area, if you have a home site; or anything else that takes up space on the acreage. But at least that gives you some sort of idea how much land you need to start with, or how many cows might fit into your program.

It also assumes the forage available is in great shape and at its optimum productivity. Pastures in the real world will rarely be in perfect shape, at least not in the early days of a new grazing plan.

Tips for Paddock Design

Paddocks should be as square as possible. This will allow the cows to spread out and not bunch at one end or the other.

Paddock Rotation

In this example, the pond needed to be fenced off to spare the banks from being damaged by cattle hooves, and so it is unavailable as a water source. The farmer created an alleyway between his paddocks and plans to haul water to their water tanks. In the winter, he will move the cattle to a sacrifice area near the barn, where his access to water is.

He has five semi- permanent larger paddocks, each with a large water tank. As his grazing plan develops, he's going to try using temporary electric fence to further subdivide them, radiating out from the water tank in each paddock. He knows he will get some compaction of the soil at the water tanks.

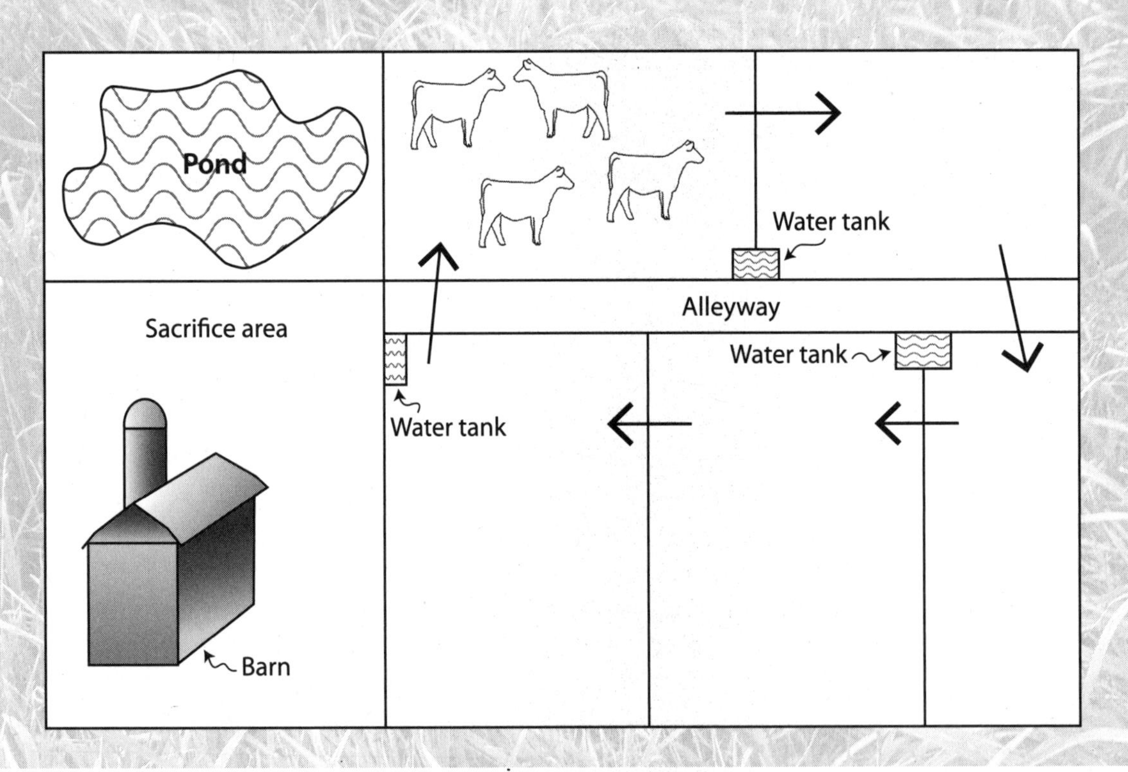

Research has shown that cows don't like to get more than 800 feet from water. If the paddock is long and skinny with the water at one end, they will make more use of the forages close to the water.

How big is an acre?

An acre is 43,560 square feet. It's hard for me to visualize a number like that, and one of the best metaphors I've ever found is to think of an acre as 75% of an American football field, or as pretty much the same as a football field with the end zones lopped off.

An acre, as a unit of measure, was defined as the amount of land a man and an ox could plow in a day. OK, that measure is great but it doesn't tell me what time the man got out of bed and began his day, or what type of ox team he had… if they were quick-footed Milking Devons, that measure might be much larger!

Rotational grazing, done properly, is the best tool for regenerating pastures, maximizing forage production, and keeping animals healthy.

It's not an overnight process, though. It will take a bit of time for you to get a feel for the rate of regrowth and how fast, or how slowly, you will be able to move your cattle through the paddocks. Expect to get it wrong a few times in the initial endeavor. It also may take a year or two to begin to see benefits. Stick with it. Try new things, tweak your strategy, and start again each grazing season with optimism. You're investing for the long term, for your pasture, your livestock, and ultimately, the environment.

---

6 "Back to Grass: The Market Potential for U.S. Grassfed Beef," Stone Barns Center for Food & Agriculture, April 2017, pg. 6, https://pastureproject.org/publications/back-to-grass-the-market-potential-for-u-s-grassfed-beef/

Glossary

- **Abomasum**
  True stomach of the cow's digestive system, performs digestive activity.
- **Allantois**
  Membranes and fluids surrounding the placenta and fetus
- **Amnion**
  Membrane and fluid surrounding the fetus
- **Bull**
  Intact male bovine
- **Castrate**
  Surgically remove testicles from male cattle
- **Colostrum**
  First milk a cow produces, high in antibodies and energy. Essential for calf survival.
- **Crossbred**
  A calf that has parents that are two different breeds
- **Dam**
  Female, used often in discussing pedigrees
- **Estrous**
  The entire heat cycle
- **Estrus**
  The period of receptivity to the male
- **Heifer**
  A young female bovine that has not had a calf yet
- **Mastitis**
  Inflammation and infection of the mammary tissue
- **Omasum**
  Part of the digestive system, functions to absorb water from feed as it is digested
- **Polled**
  A bovine that is born naturally without horns
- **Reticulum**
  A fold in the rumen
- **Rumen**
  The largest part of the cow's stomach, performs fermentation and breakdown of feeds and forage
- **Stanchion**
  A headgate or restraint that holds a cow still for milking
- **Steer**
  A castrated male bovine

Additional Reading

Temple Grandin's Guide to Working with Farm Animals
TEMPLE GRANDIN
This should be required reading for ANYONE with livestock.

The Art and Science of Grazing
SARAH FLACK
Great detailed information on grazing.

The Drought Resilient Farm
DALE STRICKLER
Lots of info on setting up water systems.

Grassfed Cattle
JULIUS REUCHEL
Lots of info on rotational grazing and the economics of a beef cattle operation.

Managing Pasture
DALE STRICKLER
Great resource for improving pasture and setting up grazing systems.

The Ethical Meat Handbook - 2nd Edition
MEREDITH LEIGH
Award-winning book about home processing and charcuterie of meat.

The Grassfed Gourmet Fires it Up!
RITA CALVERT AND MICHAEL HELLER
Cooking grassfed beef is different! Lots of info on how to cook it and a ton of recipes.

Cows Save the Planet
JUDITH D. SCHWARTZ
Info on grazing and how it can positively impact climate change.

Sacred Cow
DIANA RODGERS, RD AND ROBB WOLF
One of the best, balanced, well-researched books I've ever read regarding why well-raised beef is good for you.

Defending Beef
NICOLETTE HAHN NIEMAN
The original and one of the best books on, well... defending beef.

Index

ABOUT NEW SOCIETY PUBLISHERS

New Society Publishers is an activist, solutions-oriented publisher focused on publishing books for a world of change. Our books offer tips, tools, and insights from leading experts in sustainable building, homesteading, climate change, environment, conscientious commerce, renewable energy, and more—positive solutions for troubled times.

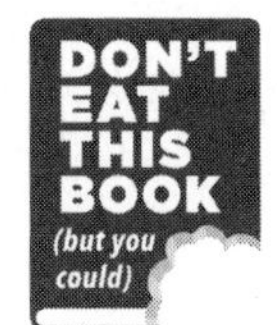

We're proud to hold to the highest environmental and social standards of any publisher in North America. When you buy New Society books, you are part of the solution!

- We print all our books in North America, never overseas.
- All our books are printed on 100% **post-consumer recycled paper**, processed chlorine-free, with low-VOC vegetable-based inks (since 2002).
- Our corporate structure is an innovative employee shareholder agreement, so we're one-third employee-owned (since 2015).
- We're carbon-neutral (since 2006).
- We're certified as a B Corporation (since 2016).
- We're Signatories to the UN's Sustainable Development Goals (SDG) Publishers Compact (2020–2030, the Decade of Action).

At New Society Publishers, we care deeply about *what* we publish—but also about *how* we do business.

To download our full catalog, please visit newsociety.com/pages/nsp-catalogue.

Sign up for New Society Publishers' newsletter for information on upcoming titles, special offers, and author events (https://signup.e2ma.net/signup/1425175/42152/).

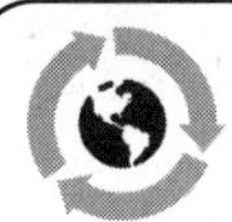

ENVIRONMENTAL BENEFITS STATEMENT

New Society Publishers saved the following resources by printing the pages of this book on chlorine free paper made with 100% post-consumer waste.

TREES	WATER	ENERGY	SOLID WASTE	GREENHOUSE GASES
35 FULLY GROWN	2,900 GALLONS	15 MILLION BTUs	120 POUNDS	15,300 POUNDS

Environmental impact estimates were made using the Environmental Paper Network Paper Calculator 4.0. For more information visit www.papercalculator.org.

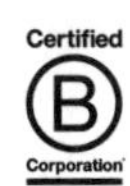

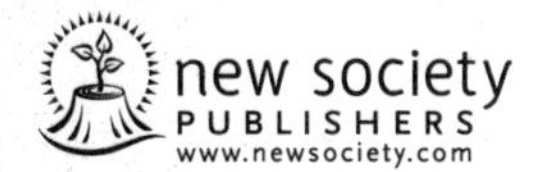

About the Authors

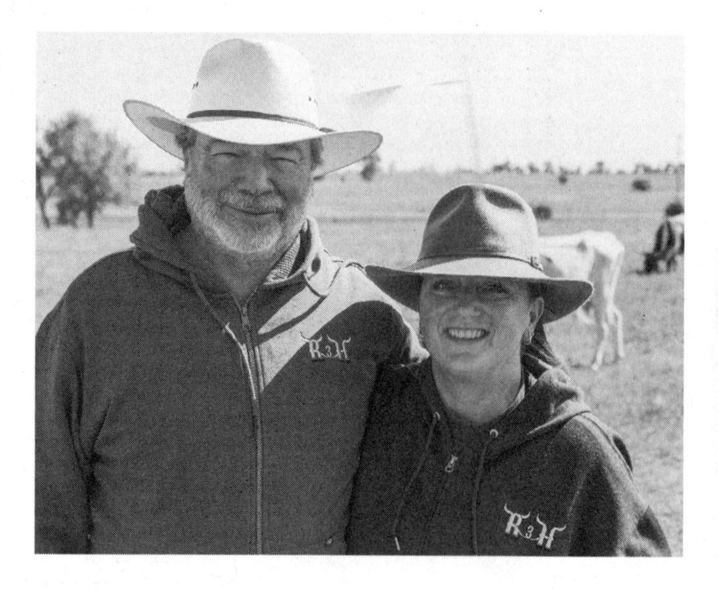

Callene and Eric Rapp have owned and operated the award-winning Rare Hare Barn since 2005, the largest heritage-breed meat-rabbit enterprise in the United States. In addition to their conservation work with rabbits, they have a large herd of heritage-breed Pineywoods cattle, and they work with the critically endangered Palmer-Dunn strain. Callene has also worked with a variety of cattle breeds at the Sedgwick County Zoo, and Eric has had experience with his family's own cow-calf operation. They have over 50 years of combined experience handling nearly every species of domestic livestock and are active members of the Livestock Conservancy. Callene is also a regular contributor to *Grit Magazine*. Authors of *Raising Rabbits for Meat*, they live and farm in Leon, Kansas.